HEARING AIDS
Current Developments and Concepts

HEARING AIDS
Current Developments and Concepts

Edited by

Martha Rubin, Ed.D.

Director, Lexington Hearing Center
Lexington School for the Deaf
New York, New York

Ardell E. Olson

University Park Press
Baltimore · London · Tokyo

UNIVERSITY PARK PRESS
International Publishers in Science and Medicine
Chamber of Commerce Building
Baltimore, Maryland 21202

Copyright © 1976 by University Park Press

Typeset by The Composing Room of Michigan, Inc.
Manufactured in the United States of America by Universal Lithographers,
Inc., and The Maple Press Co.

Library of Congress Cataloging in Publication Data
Main entry under title:
Hearing aids.
Based on the proceedings of a conference held at
the Lexington School for the Deaf, Jackson Heights,
N.Y., May 16–17, 1975.
Bibliography: p.
Includes index.
1. Hearing aids—Congresses. 2. Hearing aids—
Standards—Congresses. 3. Hearing disorders in
children—Congresses. 4. Hearing aids—Testing—
Congresses. I. Rubin, Martha. II. Lexington
School for the Deaf, New York. [DNLM: 1. Hearing
aids—Congresses. WV274 H435 1975]
RF300.H4   617.8'9   76-10623
ISBN 0-8391-0939-3

CONTENTS

Appendix A

Appendix B

CONTRIBUTORS

G. Donald Causey, Ph.D.
Chief, Central Audiology and
  Speech Pathology Program
Veterans Administration Hospital
Washington, D. C.

Leo G. Doerfler, Ph.D.
Director, Department of Audiology
The University of Pittsburgh School
  of Medicine
Eye and Ear Hospital
Pittsburgh, Pennsylvania

Rita B. Eisenberg, Sc.D.
Director, Bioacoustic Laboratory
Research Institute
St. Joseph's Hospital
Lancaster, Pennsylvania

Hubert L. Gerstman, Ph.D.
Clinical Director, Speech, Hearing
  and Language Center
New England Medical Center
  Hospital
Boston, Massachusetts

Leahea F. Grammatico, M.A.
Director, Peninsula Oral School
Redwood City, California

Edward J. Hardick, Ph.D.
Department of Audiology
Wayne State University School of
  Medicine
Detroit, Michigan

J. Donald Harris, Ph.D.
Editor, *Journal of Auditory
  Research*
Submarine Naval Base
Groton, Connecticut

Harry Levitt, Ph.D.
Communication Science
  Laboratory
Graduate Center, City University of
  New York
New York, New York

Geary A. McCandless, Ph.D.
University of Utah Medical Center
Salt Lake City, Utah

Jane R. Madell, Ph.D.
Director of Audiology Services
New York League for the Hard of
  Hearing
New York, New York

Wayne O. Olsen, Ph.D.
Otorhinolaryngology and
  Audiology
Mayo Clinic
Rochester, Minnesota

Steffi B. Resnick, Ph.D.
Communication Science
  Laboratory
Graduate Center, City University of
  New York
New York, New York

Mark Ross, Ph.D.
Department of Audiology
The University of Connecticut
Storrs, Connecticut

Martha Rubin, Ed.D.
Director, Lexington Hearing Center
Lexington School for the Deaf
New York, New York

John C. Sinclair, Ph.D.
Director of Engineering
Zenith Hearing Aid Corporation
Chicago, Illinois

Edgar Villchur, M.S.
Foundation for Hearing Aid
  Research
Woodstock, New York

Richard E. C. White, Ph.D.
Communication Science
  Laboratory
Graduate Center, City University of
  New York
New York, New York

Laura Ann Wilber, Ph.D.
Professor of Audiology
Albert Einstein College of Medicine
  of Yeshiva University
New York, New York

Annette Zaner, Ph.D.
Director of Communication
  Disorders
Mount Carmel Guild Division
Newark, New Jersey

PREFACE

This conference, which was held in May 1975, was the second of a series held at the Lexington School for the Deaf. The proceedings of this conference embody the papers of a distinguished group of audiologists, engineers, and educators as well as their spirited interactions. The conference was prompted by a need to consider the major changes in amplification within the past decade and, secondly, to consider the effect of those changes upon the hearing-impaired individual and upon the professionals involved. Those changes include: (1) the governmental enactment of performance standards and industry enactment of measurement standards for hearing aids; (2) new developments in delivery sources for children and adults; (3) the technological expertise in the measurement and recommendation of electroacoustical devices for the hearing impaired. Accordingly, a group of experts set out to discuss these issues.

The program was divided into four areas of interest: Current Developments, Standards for Electroacoustical Amplification, Hearing Aid Evaluation Procedures, and Hearing Aids for Infants and Children. These areas were selected by this writer in consultation with Dr. Mark Ross, then Director of the Willie Ross School for the Deaf, Longmeadow, Massachusetts and currently with the University of Connecticut, and also with Mr. Robert Guinta of Guinta Associates, representing industry. It was decided that there would be a panel for each of the four topics. Each panel consisted of three to five speakers, each of whom presented a formal paper. The papers occupied the first hour of each area conference and were followed by round table discussions. Thereafter, questions from the floor were discussed both by the panel and by members of the audience which was composed of health professionals.

In the afternoon session, each area conference chairperson presented the highlights of the morning meeting to a general assembly. A round table discussion adroitly conducted by Dr. Mark Ross became the final session for the day's events.

These proceedings were developed in several stages. Formal papers were reviewed by their authors for publication. The discussions were typed, and then a packet of formal papers and discussions was forwarded to the four chairpersons for editing. First names were used to preserve the informality of the sessions. In addition, each chairperson was asked to provide an introduction to his section as he saw fit. We are indebted to the four chairpersons who performed this task, namely, Dr. J. Donald Harris, Dr. Laura Wilber, Dr. Martha Rubin, and Dr. Mark Ross, who are listed in lexicon order.

When the manuscript was completed, Dr. Rita Eisenberg, a noted researcher and member of the Advisory Panel on the Review of Ear, Nose, and Throat Devices for the Food and Drug Administration, consented to provide a critique of the text and a philosophical review of hearing aid developments in an introductory chapter. A final chapter entitled "Future Perspectives" was contributed by an eminent colleague, Dr. Leo Doerfler, who attended the conference as an observer. Dr. Doerfler was awarded the Honors of the American Speech and Hearing Association in 1975 and is a past president of that Association.

Many of the day-to-day expenses of the conference and subsequent proceedings were underwritten by the Lexington School's Board of Trustees and authorized by its Executive Director, Dr. Leo E. Connor. Travel expenses of some of the participants were absorbed by friends in industry whose support helped to make the conference possible. Major industry contributors were: Audiotone Division of Royal Industries, Beltone Electronic Corporation, Bioacoustics Inc., Danavox, Inc., Guinta Associates, Precision Acoustics, Qualitone Company, Norelco of North American Phillips Company, and Zenith Hearing Instrument Corporation. Industry associate contributors were Brüel and Kjaer Precision Instruments, Oticon Corporation, and Widex Hearing Aid Company, Inc.

Valuable time was contributed by four recorders and a resource coordinator. Among this group were four certified audiologists: Ms. Marcia Rubin, Ms. Jane Brunved, Ms. Mary Jo Osberger, and Ms. Tina Jupiter, as well as a well-known educator of the deaf, Ms. Eleanor Vorce. The conference secretary, Ms. Margaret Bos, was involved in all aspects of the subsequent manuscript. Thanks are due to Ms. Barbara Hantin for her excellent typing of the actual text.

These proceedings have value for a variety of health professionals who are interested in the manufacture, delivery, and evaluation of amplification for the hearing-impaired individual in today's world.

Martha Rubin, Ed.D.

INTRODUCTION

Rita B. Eisenberg

Hearing impairment is one of the most prevalent chronic conditions in the United States (Perrin, 1975) and there is good reason to suppose that the incidence of nerve loss in the general population may be on the increase (Meyer, 1975; Schein and Delk, 1974). Further, since there is no reason at present to believe that cochlear implants and related surgical interventions for correcting or ameliorating sensorineural problems can be perfected in short order (Tonndorf, 1975), it can be expected that the number of hearing aid candidates will continue to increase substantially during coming years. Accordingly, the time has come—and, indeed, it is long past due—to take a hard look at the current hearing aid scene in order to evaluate critically what is being done by the several groups who are concerned, in one way or another, with such developments.

This volume contains the unexpurgated and frequently iconoclastic views of diverse contributors who are recognized authorities in their special fields. It covers almost all of the links in the hearing aid delivery system and airs a number of controversial issues that many professionals perhaps might prefer to sweep under the rug. It is, in other words, a healthy exercise in self-criticism that, thoughtfully evaluated, may suggest paths to badly needed improvements in services to the hearing impaired.

There is no question that hearing aids, like many other things in our technologically oriented society, have changed dramatically within the past half century and particularly within the past decade. The "big box" body aid of not so long ago, like the ear trumpet, has become a curiosity. Amplifiers now can be fitted into the temples of eyeglass frames or attached inconspicuously behind the ear. It has become possible to amplify sound in both ears rather than only in one and to aid the young infant as well as the adult.

Unfortunately, technological change has not done away with the large variety of problems that hearing aids present. How should aids be designed to yield maximum benefits to a hearing impaired population that encompasses numerous etiologies, differing audiometric patterns, and almost the entire span of human life? What kinds of standardized measurements can assure that a given model of hearing aid manufactured by a given company is uniform with others in its class or that all models of aids meet certain minimal standards? Who shall make such determinations and who shall enforce them? Are the most commonly used methods for predicting the benefits of hearing aid use and assessing the merits of selected models the best methods? And, if they are not, what alternatives now are available? What kind of distribution system best can serve the needs of the hearing impaired? What kinds of supportive services are required?

These are some of the important questions to which this book is addressed and none is susceptible to simplistic answers. There are honest disagreements among experts, partly because of differences in background, but mainly because of state-of-the-art problems that have triggered widespread activity among professional, governmental, industrial, and consumer groups.[1] Such problems are common in any area that is changing rapidly and, in this Introduction, it perhaps might be useful to emphasize certain issues that are especially significant.

A major problem underlying many of the present difficulties is that recent advances in technology have not been accompanied by any landmark advances in our knowledge about how the human auditory system works under pathological conditions—or, for that matter, even under normal conditions. Indeed, current thinking in the area of auditory physiology is in flux and, in the absence of adequate substantive information, little of the deluge of new data is immediately applicable to hearing aid design or selection procedures. Hearing aids, despite advances, remain essentially amplifiers and standardized hearing aid selection procedures remain essentially those set forth by Carhart back in 1946.

Another problem is a failure to deal properly with the fact that the population of hearing aid users has changed drastically since audiology emerged as a discipline in the 1940's. New case finding techniques have led to the aiding of very young infants whose auditory processing abilities are very largely unknown and, consequently, untestable in routine ways. The conquest of disease has led to increased survival rates among the elderly,

[1] Groups that have been especially active include:
(a) *Professional:* American Academy of Rehabilitative Audiology; American Council of Otolaryngology; American National Standards Association (ANSI), S3-48 Working Group (chaired by Samuel Lybarger); American Speech and Hearing Association.
(b) *Governmental:* Bureau of Medical Devices and Diagnostic Products, Food and Drug Administration; Environmental Protection Agency; Federal Trade Commission; Intradepartmental Task Force on Hearing Aids, Dept. of H.E.W.; National Institute of Neurologic and Communicative Disorders and Stroke; permanent Subcommittee on Investigation, chaired by Senator Ribicoff; Small Business Committee on Government Regulation, chaired by Senator McIntire; Subcommittee on Consumer Interests of the Elderly, chaired by Senator Church.
(c) *Industrial:* Greater Philadelphia Hearing Aid Dealers Guild; Hearing Aid Industry Conference (HAIC); National Association of Earmold Laboratories; National Hearing Aid Society (NHAS).
(d) *Consumer:* Retired Professional Action Group (Gray Panthers); Vermont Public Interest Research Group.

Table 1. Percentage of significant bilateral hearing impairment by age

Age in years	Percent of total population, 1971[1]
Under 6	0.8
6–16	5.9 (6.4)
17–24	3.6
25–44	9.8
45–64	28.6
65–and over	51.3

Extrapolated from Schein and Delk, 1974, p. 29.
[1] N = 6,549,643.

many of whom are subject to poorly understood processing disorders in addition to diminished hearing acuity.

Although it is impossible to come up with exact figures on the age characteristics of today's hearing aid users, it is relatively easy to arrive at reliable estimates by extrapolating from independently obtained data compilations. As a case in point, Tables 1, 2, and 3 give percentage and rate values derived by the National Census for the Deaf Population (Table 1), Zenith Radio Corporation (Table 2), and the National Center for Health Statistics (Table 3). They represent, in order, the proportion of those with substantial binaural hearing loss, the proportion of those who have purchased hearing aids from a representative manufacturer within the past five years, and the rate per thousand population of those reporting hearing aid use in 1971 as well as twelve years earlier. As can be seen, each of these different sources yields strikingly similar information: the bulk of the hearing aid candidate population falls into the 65-years-or-over category and, judging by Table 3, the rate is increasing.

Let us consider, then, some further characteristics of this very large group of elderly hearing aid users. According to Perrin (1975), close to half of them have family incomes of $5,000 or less per year and less than 10% of them have incomes of $15,000 or more. More than 60% of them have additional chronic disabilities that sharply limit their ability to shop

Table 2. Percentage of hearing aid purchasers by age

Age in years	Percent of total hearing aid sales
Under 11	6.5
12–24	4.2
25–49	9.0
50–65	24.0
65–and over	56.5

Extrapolated from 1970–1975 warrantee information provided by Zenith Radio Corporation.

Table 3. Number of noninstitutionalized persons with hearing aids
and number per 1,000 population by age: United States, July
1958–June 1959 and 1971

Age in years	Persons with hearing aids			
	July 1958–June 1959	1971[1]	July 1958–June 1959	1971
	Number in thousands		Number per 1,000 persons	
(All ages)	(1,162)	(1,695)	(6.8)	(8.8)
Under 45	156	224	1.3	1.7
45–64	358	436	10.2	10.4
65–and over	648	1,035	43.7	53.5

Unpublished data from the Health Interview Survey, National Center
for Health Statistics.
Data are based on household interviews of the civilian population.
[1] Excludes persons under 3 years of age.

around for purposes of diagnostic evaluation or hearing aid selection.[2] A
substantial proportion of them live at some distance from population
centers where diagnostic and rehabilitative services most easily were available. More than half of them have eight or fewer years of formal education.

Generalizing from these data, then, it must be recognized that a
majority of hearing aid candidates are: (1) elderly; (2) poor; (3) saddled
with other health problems that make travel difficult and, in some cases,
impossible; (4) located inconveniently far from metropolitan service
facilities; and (5) relatively uneducated. (HEW Report, 1975).

Let us turn now to the other pole of the age continuum and consider
what the situation is with respect to infants and preschoolers who are
hearing aid candidates. Although they constitute a very small proportion
of all candidates (see Tables), they also have very special needs which, in
most cases, raise the costs of both diagnostic and rehabilitative services.
The younger they are, the more exacting and time consuming are the
special procedures required for evaluating their hearing abilities and selecting aids with suitable characteristics. A majority of them will be lifetime
hearing aid users and, as development proceeds and characteristics of the
external canal change, they must be supplied with new earmolds at regular
intervals. They cannot be expected to show any discretion in caring for
hearing aids themselves and, since their instruments almost invariably will
be worn during active play as well as under less stressful conditions, a high

[2] The association between hearing impairment and other chronic disabilities is not
confined to the elderly: the Office of Demographic Studies at Gallaudet College has
reported that about one third of all students attending special education programs are
multiply handicapped (Perrin, 1975).

rate of hearing aid breakdown is predictable. From a management stand-point, then, it is mandatory that spare aids, spare parts, and speedy repair services be available for them.

Using only these two poles of the age continuum as our indicators, one finds facts that have implications for almost every aspect of the hearing aid manufacture and delivery system:

First, they suggest that hearing aids must be hardy. That is to say, instruments must stand up under a variety of atmospheric and usage conditions and require a minimum of care and servicing.

Second, they suggest that aids must be so designed as to permit *easy* manipulation and regulation of such parts as gain and frequency controls. The minuscule gain controls on today's ear level aids, which are frequently unmarked and almost invariably lacking in detents or even such tactile cues as raised areas to indicate halfway amplification points, almost defy the efforts of arthritic fingers to set volume at comfort level. Frequency controls, which more often are found inside the case rather than outside, are guaranteed to make adjustments difficult.

Third, they suggest that efforts somehow must be made to hold down the purchase price of aids (which now range roughly from two hundred dollars to upwards of four hundred dollars).[3]

Fourth, they suggest that an effective evaluation and distribution system must take into account those hearing aid candidates who, for one reason or another, cannot be accommodated within traditional outpatient evaluation facilities or by very widely dispersed repair facilities.

Finally, they suggest that those who, by reason of limited education or sophistication, are unable to protect themselves from the unscrupulous, must be safeguarded by suitable labeling and guarantee provisions.

It must be admitted that few of these goals can be achieved either easily or quickly. Manufacturers, for sound practical and economic rea-sons, are reluctant to change design features that have taken years to develop; and they clearly are reluctant to pool their efforts and share new or especially desirable features with competitors. Dispensers, whatever their affiliations, must base pricing policies not only upon inventory costs, but also upon the costs of whatever ancillary services they provide. Most privately supported professional groups have neither the wherewithal nor the personnel to set up mobile vans, monthly "country clinics," or related facilities whereby an outlying population of potential hearing aid users can be provided with diagnostic and hearing aid selection services,—which means that community agencies at some level must not only recognize these needs, but also provide the funding to meet them (Rower, 1976). Manufacturers and dealers alike express dissatisfaction with the idea of centralized repair stations in strategically located areas (personal communi-cations) and, as various chapters of this volume amply testify, many elements of the hearing aid distribution system are antagonistic to the idea of government-mandated testing and/or labeling procedures.

[3] According to the HEW Intradepartmental Task Force Report on Hearing Aids, September 1974: "It is well known among dealers that retail price is calculated on a multiple in excess of three times the dealer's price." (p. 40).

Government-mandated testing and labeling procedures already are in the developmental stage, however, and, at the risk of offending both contributors to this book and readers of it, I would like to suggest that, by neglecting some of the needs this book spells out, members of the hearing aid distribution chain have brought such troubles upon themselves. I additionally would like to suggest that some forms of government intervention are not entirely bad. Whatever criticisms may be leveled at the Food and Drug Administration (FDA),[4] —and various criticisms can be found within this book,—the very threat of mandatory controls has resulted in the promulgation of revised national standards for measuring the electroacoustic characteristics of hearing aids. The FDA, in effect, has acted as a catalyst and, while doing so, has benefitted greatly by accepting almost in toto realistic procedures that already were being considered and/or used by reputable organizations at various levels of the distribution system.

Some of the standards perhaps may be debatable, but there is nothing in FDA bylaws to prevent amending them as experience dictates or new information is obtained. It must be recognized that the purpose of mandatory standards is to obtain compliance from a minority of manufacturers who refuse to comply with self-imposed industry standards without hamstringing the majority of manufacturers who maintain voluntary controls. It already has been conceded that such a recalcitrant minority, in fact, does exist (Sinclair, 1974); and it is the express function of the FDA, as the consumer's voice in Washington, D.C., to assure that devices are safe and effective.

It is worth noting that the American Speech and Hearing Association (ASHA), as well as industry, dealer, and consumer groups, offered advice and some practical assistance during the long period when problems of setting hearing aid standards were being considered by the FDA. Advice was offered by ASHA in two significant areas: lack of product uniformity and lack of product reliability. ASHA, however, had no real position on defining performance characteristics for a hearing aid standard (McLaughlin, 1975). This seems an extraordinary state of affairs when an organization has so many members so heavily involved with the hearing impaired.[5]

[4] Food and Drug Administration
Bureau of Medical Devices and Diagnostic Products
Div. of Classif. & Scientific Eval. (HFK-4)
Panel on Review of Ear, Nose, and Throat Devices 1975 Membership List: Harry W. McCurdy, M.D.—Chairman, Rita B. Eisenberg, Sc.D., James Jerger, Ph.D., Jean L. McCarrey—Consumer Representative, Walter C. McLean, M.D., Arthur F. Niemoeller, D.Sc., Harry Sauberman—Executive Secretary, F. Blair Simmons, M.D., Russell L. Thompson—Industry Representative, and, Gabriel F. Tucker, Jr. M.D.

[5] Editor's Note: As the Introduction indicates, some of the comments made in these proceedings are critical of ASHA. It is the editor's concern that this fact may be construed as representative of a situation in which there was no opportunity for comment or clarification by ASHA. Unfortunately, the Associate Secretary for Audiology, who had accepted an invitation to attend the conference, could not attend becasue of an ASHA Executive Board meeting. The alternate he suggested was also unable to attend.

It is my feeling that ASHA cannot much longer avoid concern with such issues. Moreover, it may be time for the organization to assert leadership in other important areas, specifically those relating to curriculum development, more adequate funding for research pertaining to hearing aid evaluation and use, and with the dissemination of information that is helpful to suppliers, regulatory agencies, and the public at large. Despite the complexities of today's hearing aids, many major universities offer little or no coursework on their technical aspects, the effects of vented versus closed earmolds, or the problems associated with calibration under differing conditions. Research funds need to be lobbied for if new programs in all areas pertaining to hearing aid use are to be developed. Guidelines for labeling, based upon the clinical experience of ASHA members, should be made available to manufacturers, to appropriate federal agencies, and to the general public. In short, ASHA might do well to reconsider its priorities and assume a positive and highly visible stance with respect to current issues. The contents of this book suggest what some of those priorities might be.

LITERATURE CITED

Carhart, R. 1946. Tests for selection of hearing aids. Laryngoscope 56:780–794.

Dept. of Health, Education and Welfare. Final Report to the Secretary on Hearing Health Care, July 1975.

McLaughlin, R. N. 1975. Report to the Ear, Nose and Throat Panel of the Food and Drug Administration, June 30, 1975.

Meyer, A. F. 1975. Report of the Environmental Protection Agency, presented to the Ear, Nose and Throat Panel of the Food and Drug Administration, June 30, 1975.

Perrin, E. B. 1975. Statement before the Subcommittee on Government Regulation: U. S. Senate Select Committee on Small Business, May 20, 1975.

Rower, M. C. 1976. Identification audiometry on the move. Aud. Hear. Educ. 2:13–15.

Schein, J. D., and Delk, M. T. Jr. 1974. The Deaf Population of United States. Natl. Assn. of the Deaf, Silver Springs, Md.

Sinclair, J. 1974. Report to the Ear, Nose and Throat Panel of the Food and Drug Administration, December 9, 1974.

Tonndorf, J. 1975. Report to the Ear, Nose and Throat Panel of the Food and Drug Administration, December 1, 1975.

HEARING AIDS
Current Developments and Concepts

CURRENT
DEVELOPMENTS
IN
HEARING
AIDS

INTRODUCTION

J. Donald Harris

Probably no electronic gadget of our gadget-ridden society has suffered as many adjustments as the hearing aid. About every 5 years a complete revolution is accomplished: the microphone changes drastically, whole new circuits are devised, the earpiece is entirely new, and new concepts are validated for mating the instrument to the person's ear(s). A hearing aid dispenser must continuously revise his knowledge or risk being almost hopelessly outdated. Audiology schools, clinics, and centers must continuously introduce newer components and models to keep up with the latest prostheses and techniques.

Fortunately, though, the hearing aid industry is so well self-advised in the fields of electronics and plastics that each generation of hearing aids outperforms the former by a couple of light years. Gain and maximum power output are way up even in small models, distortion is way down, frequencies extend further both up and down by octaves, peaks are smoothed, and a wide variety of adjustments and earpiece components is available to allow tailoring the total prosthesis to the patient's needs and capabilities with a nicety hitherto only dreamed. Not so long ago, the fantastic suggestion was being made that one hearing aid would not only serve all patients, but serve all patients best! Today a bewildering array of components and entire units, and the whole CROS family, are at the dispenser's fingertips, and the notion of a single "best" system has been abandoned. Today the industry offers ear-level instruments for the severely deaf; log compression for the recruiting ear; adaptations for the elderly, the monaurally defective, the high-tone hypacusic; and even units adaptable to babes before their first babble, so that scores of thousands are suitable candidates where before an aid profited them naught.

But while the industry and the hearing health delivery team generally can take real pride in the situation now as compared with only a few years ago, there remains a large area for improvement. Major steps are still to be taken in both hardware and software.

As to hardware, in the not-too-distant future are aids which tamper with timing and frequency as well as with amplitude, and which otherwise process speech so as to ungarble it for the presbycusic ear, so that the patient with central nervous system involvement, atherosclerosis, etc., and many more thousands will become good candidates for the creative dispenser.

As to software, really major changes, quite as important as those in hardware, must be developed and standardized for optimum results. In this phase the experimental audiologist should take the lead. I think of four general areas:

RELATIONSHIP BETWEEN ELECTROACOUSTIC CHARACTERISTICS OF AN AID AND VALIDATED USER PERFORMANCE TESTS

Only a handful of centers have a true artificial ear or artificial head necessary to determine, with the breadth and precision demanded today, the electroacoustical performance of an aid. There is no standard way to quantify the extremely important variables of intermodulation and transient distortion in aids, although there are encouraging attempts. Identification of attack and release times and of variable input/output ratios cannot be done well without expensive arrays; determining the directional response of an aid demands an anechoic chamber. In short, the day is long past (about 3 years!) when a clinic with a sound level meter and a 2-cc coupler can pretend it has explored the physical properties of an aid.

Presently, many places are trying hard to upgrade their facilities so that they can adequately characterize the physical properties of every aid in their stock. This is not only a foolhardy cost in personnel and material, it is, strictly speaking, the responsibility of the manufacturer, whose measurement methods and quality control should be carefully monitored by the industry. One looks forward to the day when the manufacturer furnishes, with every aid, standardized engineering information that the dispenser, on the basis of a broad body of behavioral research, is known to require. It is this research that the audiologist should provide.

DETERMINATION OF CANDIDACY FOR AN AID

The psychoacoustic testing of a client to determine whether he or she is likely to profit from a prosthesis, and by how much, is still a wide-open field. Even if one concentrates on speech reception to the exclusion of everything else our ears do for us, it cannot be said that we have a standard method of assessment. We do not even know what speech test to use or whether to degrade it with white noise, pink noise, speech-like noise, Babelic noise, or with a competing message. Of the many ways to degrade speech besides adding noise, not one has been seriously adapted to aid evaluation.

DETERMINATION OF AIDED PERFORMANCE

Even if one has a good candidate and the theoretically ideal prosthesis for him, there is no validated way to measure, much less to predict, what that aid does in the wearer's daily life. Without such research and validated evaluation, the audiologist today is in no position to state on any basis other than his "clinical judgment," however good that may be, which aid is best for his client and how much good it will do. To state otherwise is to arrogate to the audiologist a level of objectivity and scientific caution which is not apparent to the scientist.

It is known that an unaided versus aided test with a few phonetically balanced word lists is hopelessly inadequate, and certainly a graduate audiologist is not needed to run such a test. Most people throw up their hands and simply let the client wear the aid for a time and make up his mind. This is given the cloak of respectability by using jargon like "client-oriented evaluation." This may be the only evaluation possible given the present state of audiological knowledge, and I do not deny that patients in many cases may be well served, but it is to be laughed out of court as in any way a scientific or even economical procedure. If this is all one could hope for, audiologists should indeed throw up not only their hands but also their lunch.

If there were, on the other hand, a battery of tests which a trained person could use to measure performance in a variety of user situations, the optimum aid could be identified with reasonable celerity and the long drawn-out "trial period" of days and even weeks for each possible aid be drastically shortened or, ideally, eliminated. Present research here should be accelerated many-fold.

CONTINUED OPTIMUM USE OF AID BY PATIENT

Surveys show that, not only in the general population, but also in facilities where an aid should play an even more vital role (such as schools and classes for the hearing impaired and residences for the elderly), a heavy fraction of aids is always unused for any or all of several correctable reasons. It is the audiologist's responsibility to the public to identify what these reasons are and how to correct them. He even may have to go a bit outside his professional role and act as a sort of individual advocate. The thought is being expressed these days that the audiologist, in addition to his own rehabilitative skills, may be the most appropriate professional to help the user draw on other community resources that may be desirable and available.

In this opening section of the book, a few of these issues are discussed. Dr. Causey, who for many years has headed the widely respected research and clinical program in hearing aids for the Veterans Administration, gives an overview of today's policy and practice. Dr. Hardick, a national leader in rehabilitative audiology, presents a viewpoint on aid dispensing, and Dr. Gerstman, in the forefront of research in speech intelligibility, summarizes one of his experiments to date that promises to add significantly to the audiologist's test battery.

CURRENT DEVELOPMENTS IN HEARING AIDS

G. Donald Causey

Certainly, the most current development in the field of hearing aids has been the public attention given to hearing aids recently. The Food and Drug Administration, the Federal Trade Commission, consumer groups, and several committees on Capitol Hill have thrown the spotlight on hearing aids. Licensing activities have made battlegrounds of some state legislatures. On another front, a new measurement standard is in preparation by the American National Standards Institute; a new performance standard is being prepared at the request of the Food and Drug Administration. The Zwislocki coupler and the Knowles Electronics Manikin for Acoustic Research, known as KEMAR, have achieved a great deal of acceptance from audiologists and manufacturers as improved tools for measurement and research. The climate then reflects changes in attitudes regarding measurement, performance, distribution systems, prices, and hearing aid candidacy. With so much attention directed toward hearing aids, we can certainly anticipate developments which will benefit the hearing impaired.

CROS AND BICROS FITTINGS

In the area of hearing aids themselves, one of the most interesting developments has been the way in which the use pattern of hearing aids has

Table 1. Aids issued contract year 1975 by the Veterans Administration

Type	Number	Total issue (%)
On-the-body	2,030	14.2
Over-the-ear	5,197	36.5
Eyeglass regular	1,522	10.7
Eyeglass BICROS	638	4.5
Eyeglass CROS	1,898	13.3
High-pass	1,061	7.4
In-the-ear	346	2.4
Directional	713	5.0
Compression	747	5.2
Bone conduction eyeglass	102	0.7
	14,254	99.9

changed in recent years. For example, as Table 1 indicates, 17.8% of Veterans Administration patients last year were issued CROS or BICROS hearing aids. The staff of the Walter Reed Army Hospital in Washington issued CROS or BICROS hearing aids to 30% of their patients last year. These percentages are probably higher than the statistics from community centers and university clinics. One reason for this is that hearing aids in eyeglasses are avoided by many audiologists because of the fitting problems. These fitting problems may be minimized soon. In April 1975, representatives from the Optical Manufacturers Association and hearing aid manufacturers met to discuss improvements in the design and fitting of eyeglass aids, paving the way for the real potential of the CROS and BICROS concept to be realized. In addition, the advent of the wireless CROS hearing aid makes the fitting easier and eliminates the need to return the aid to the factory for soldering of connections. It is expected that, without wires to break, there will be reduced incidence of repair with the wireless CROS hearing aid.

DIRECTIONAL HEARING AIDS

Candidacy

Directional hearing aids continue to attract the attention of the hearing impaired. Many find that reduced amplification of signals from behind can be a hindrance rather than a blessing, and some people object to not being tuned in to everything around them. Hearing-impaired clients who are the best candidates for directional hearing aids work in fixed environments with noise emanating from the rear of their work position, such as an air conditioner installed in the window behind the desk. In clinical practice we have found it advantageous to permit the person considering the directional aid for the first time to take it with him to his home and place of employment to try it under actual conditions. A hearing aid that offers a range of attenuation of signals from behind might prove to be most beneficial for some patients.

Measurement of Directional Aids with KEMAR

Directional hearing aids require more than the usual electroacoustic measurements to evaluate their physical performance. Even adding a front-to-back signal ratio does not provide sufficient information. A front-to-back signal ratio indicates the number of decibels by which the amplification of a signal from in front of the aid exceeds the amplification of a signal from the rear of the aid. Figure 1 shows a block diagram of the equipment array. To accomplish the measurement, one identifies a test point midway between two speakers fixed at the level of KEMAR's ears. The calibration of the stimuli to be presented through the front and rear speakers is conducted with KEMAR out of the anechoic chamber. A monitor microphone at the test point permits the adjustment to 60 decibels (dB) sound

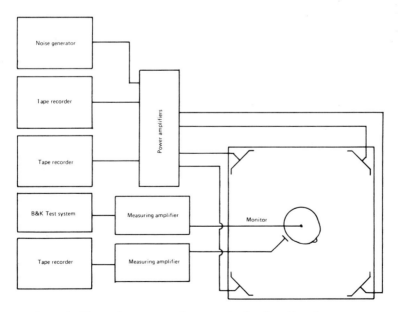

Figure 1. The equipment array for measuring hearing aid performance.

pressure level (SPL) of each test stimulus in turn. KEMAR is returned to the test point after the calibration procedure. The volume control of the hearing aid is adjusted to yield 12 dB down from saturation with a 60-dB SPL input of speech spectrum noise from the front speaker. The output of the hearing aid, measured at the coupler, is noted. With the speech spectrum noise coming from the rear speaker, in absence of other signals, a measure is made at the coupler. The front-to-back signal ratio is computed by subtracting the level produced by the signal at the rear speaker from the level produced by the signal at the front speaker.

The front-to-back signal ratio in directional hearing aids ranged from 6 dB to 19 dB with the mean around 12 dB in the sample most recently studied. One can employ speakers on the sides as well in measuring the front-to-back signal ratio. Some believe the use of several speakers would yield a more realistic ratio since noise is generally all around us. The investigator should use uncorrelated noise when making such a measurement.

Real Ear Measurement of Directional Aids

Hearing aids differ in the way in which they treat the signal from the rear. With some aids the signal from the rear is clear and conversation from the rear is easily understood, just attenuated. With other hearing aids the conversation from the rear is attenuated, but muddy and unclear. With an aid like this, patients may indeed feel tuned out and unable to react to warning signals. Therefore, in addition to the electroacoustic measurements, a test battery should include a subjective evaluation using normal and hearing-impaired listeners. With the same equipment array as indicated previously, we record the output of each directional hearing aid in the presence of our recordings of the Revised CID Sentences coming from the front speaker and a recording of continuous discourse coming from the rear speaker. Quality judgments made from these tapes assist the audiologist in making decisions in the selection of directional hearing aids for contract or for clinic stock. In the clinical evaluation of directional aids, we think the patient is better served if a competing signal is used, whether it be continuous discourse, babble, or cafeteria noise.

COMPRESSION AIDS

Measurement

In measuring compression hearing aids to determine quality, electroacoustic measurements do not tell the whole story, even when families of curves and measurement of attack and release times are added. It has been necessary to record music and speech at an input level of 80 dB through the hearing aids in order to add another dimension to the evaluation. The range of quality in the reproduction is amazing, but so is the annual improvement in compression hearing aids as manufacturers gain more experience and utilize new technology. In 1973 we studied 19 compression hearing aids, and none were found to be acceptable. Today, there is a wide variety that is clinically useful. In the clinical evaluation of compression hearing aids, it is recommended that a speech signal be included at a level that drives the aid into compression so that the patient can evaluate how well the aid controls the signal.

HIGH-PASS HEARING AIDS

Inventory

High-pass over-the-ear hearing aids comprise 7.4% of our issue. In order to satisfy the range of high frequency hearing impairments, it is necessary to have at least three such aids in one's inventory: an aid which amplifies only the frequencies above 1,000 Hertz (Hz); an aid which amplifies only those frequencies above 1,500 Hz; and an aid which amplifies only those frequencies above 2,000 Hz. Earmold and tubing adjustments are used to further enhance hearing aid performance.

Measurement of High-pass Hearing Aids

High-pass hearing aids are measured utilizing a Zwislocki coupler and KEMAR in an anechoic chamber. This allows the audiologist to demonstrate the effect of earmold acoustics together with the characteristics of the instrument, which is not possible with the 2-cc coupler. With KEMAR, however, there is difficulty in achieving a flat frequency response at the test point with the use of a monitor microphone. To handle this problem, the microphone at the Zwislocki coupler was made the monitor microphone, and a frequency response was recorded on the level recorder. At the same time, the output of the oscillator was recorded on tape. The microphone in KEMAR was then converted to a measuring microphone, and the tape-recorded signal was played synchronously with the frequency markings on the recording paper. A flat response verifies the efficacy of this technique. The sensitivity of this system to any movement of KEMAR sometimes necessitates making new test tapes each half day. The resultant hearing aid frequency response represents the orthotelephonic gain of the instrument, an indication of the sound pressure present at the eardrum.

High-pass Hearing Aids with Open Molds

To measure high-pass hearing aids using an open earmold, the volume control of the hearing aid is adjusted to a level just below acoustic feedback. The frequency response in Figure 2 is that of a high-pass hearing aid tested with an open earmold. Even though the volume control has been reduced so that there is no audible feedback, a spike which is thought to represent incipient feedback can be observed in the frequency response. The frequency responses in Figure 3 were developed to investigate incipient feedback further. The gain at 1,000 Hz was reduced 3 dB for curve B and another 3 dB for curve C. The spike disappears almost entirely with the reduction of gain. Therefore, an important recommendation is that frequency responses of high-pass aids measured with open earmolds be conducted with the volume control adjusted to a level just below audible feedback and then reduced 5 dB more in order to ensure absence of incipient feedback.

SIGNAL PROCESSING HEARING AIDS

A current development in hearing aids is the major research effort to bring totally new concepts to the field of amplification for the hearing-impaired. Hearing aids at the present time are primarily amplifiers of signals. In the future, hearing aids are going to be processors of signals, coupling the signals in better fashion to the existing hearing residual. It is quite possible for the frequency response of a hearing aid to be divided into 10 or 15 or 20 separate frequency bands, each individually tuneable without contributing distortion to the signal. Furthermore, it should be possible for hearing aids in the future to identify speech in the presence of noise and amplify only the speech signal. Research activities in areas such as these have been underway for a number of years.

COMPUTERIZED HEARING AIDS AND EVALUATIONS

Hearing aid evaluations are going to become more and more complex. Certain of the developments in hearing aid design presently underway will require the audiologist to operate a minicomputer in order to make the necessary adjustments in the aids. Although signal-processing hearing aids are in the future, audiologists must prepare for their arrival. Certainly one of the first things we can do is to break away from our conservative mold and use the various types of hearing aids presently available in the marketplace.

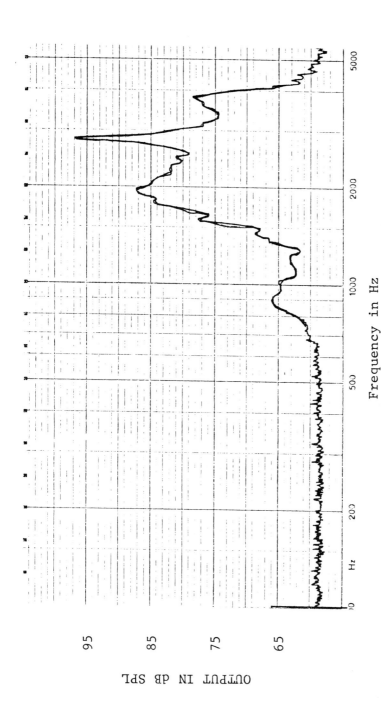

Figure 2. Orthotelephonic frequency response of a hearing aid utilizing KEMAR and an open earmold. The spike at 2,800 Hz is representative of incipient feedback.

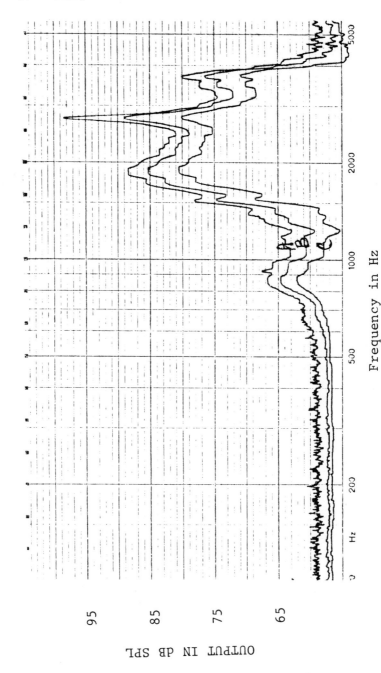

Figure 3. Orthotelephonic frequency response of a hearing aid utilizing KEMAR and an open earmold. Curves B and C represent volume control rotation to decrease gain at 1,000 Hz by 3 dB. As a result, incipient feedback is no longer present.

RECOMMENDATIONS

We must develop new speech discrimination tools and insist on complete information from the manufacturer for each of his models. We must have a heightened awareness with regard to the importance of hearing aid evaluations and a push by the American Speech and Hearing Association to insist that training institutions expand their course work in hearing aids and aural rehabilitation.

DISCUSSION

DR. HARRIS: There are many aspects of the hearing aids field in which striking developments are occurring. From my perspective of 30 years, there is ferment in the hearing health delivery services to the individual.

DIRECTIONAL HEARING AIDS

AUDIENCE MEMBER: You remarked that some long-time users of hearing aids found the directional aid different and, therefore, somewhat unpleasant. Was this experiential? Once more experience was obtained with the directional aid, did opinion change?

DR. CAUSEY: We very carefully develop with the patient an analysis of his needs and explain to him the advantages of directional aids, especially if he is working in a noisy environment. We are "fortunate" in having a very noisy cafeteria in our building where the patient can use that type of aid, together with other types of instruments. After a whole day with us with the aid(s), he has had experience in using it. There have been those who, even though warned that they must get used to the "tuning out," did return within a couple of weeks and say that they could not get used to it. However, not many return the instrument, primarily because they have spent enough time with it to know its advantages and disadvantages and, secondly, because we have discussed the aid and how it works in some depth with each patient.

SPARE HEARING AIDS

AUDIENCE MEMBER: What is the use of directional aids for children, especially in classrooms?

DR. CAUSEY: I haven't worked with children except to a very small degree. Nonetheless, one shouldn't treat hearing aids as is often done. For example, I have three or four pairs of eyeglasses. I would like to see the day when each user has two or three hearing aids, among which would be a directional type and a regular type. Then, when the newer aid needs repair, one has a spare to fall back upon.

DR. HARRIS: Then the reason for the second aid would be not only as a spare, but for quite different purposes. Is there some way of having this flexibility built into the present aid?

DR. CAUSEY: There are some on the market with that capability and they do work.

VETERANS ADMINISTRATION DATA PUBLICATION

DR. CAUSEY: The Veterans Administration (V.A.) has taken a very low profile on hearing aids and is being forced more and more, by the emphasis of consumer groups and also by the Freedom of Information Act, to publish the information that it generates on aids. In 1976, the V. A. data published on hearing aids will probably be double that of the previous year. The Government Printing Office will have released "A Handbook of Hearing Aid Information—1976," containing, for all directional aids, message-competition ratios of two types, polar coordinates, and the usual other information. There will be much more information than ever before.

V. A. CLINICAL PROCEDURES

DR. DOERFLER: There are standardized procedures in the V. A. for making certain kinds of electroacoustic measurements upon which purchasing is based. Do you have, or want, a comparable set of standardized procedures at the level of your clinical facilities?

DR. CAUSEY: I am all for standardization, but at the moment I do not have a clinical procedure. The clinical procedures are all still experimental. We have developed materials, not yet available to all of our own clinics, which we employ to evaluate these aids clinically.

DR. DOERFLER: What are the comparabilities in the procedures in your clinic? In your records do you find different patterns of distribution for various clinics since they use different approaches?

DR. CAUSEY: There are different issue rates depending upon the clinic. Some are more interested in this feature, some in that. We have 46 clinics evaluating and issuing aids, and we probably have 46 different methods for doing it.

V. A. ELECTROACOUSTIC ANALYSIS OF AIDS

AUDIENCE MEMBER: Do you test every aid acoustically before you issue it?

DR. CAUSEY: Last year we did not. This year our clinicians have a frequency response from our own distribution center on every aid they dispense. The purpose of this frequency response is not just for the clinician but also for the instrument when it requires repair. The frequency response, once the aid is issued, goes along with the aid back to the repair center. Then when the aid comes back from repair, we can be sure that it is as good as new.

AUDIENCE MEMBER: How do you do these initial measurements? How do you set up a test situation for the aid?

DR. CAUSEY: We use the larger Brüel and Kjaer test chamber (about 4 feet on a side) using regular Brüel and Kjaer equipment. To select aids for contract, they are evaluated in two places—at the National Bureau of Standards using a small chamber and at the University of Maryland using the larger chamber. We make all the regular types of measurement and some special ones.

DEFECTIVE HEARING AIDS

AUDIENCE MEMBER: We recently started purchasing aids and checking every aid that came into the clinic. We found that the specification sheets from the manufacturer did not agree with our tests. When we called the manufacturer, we were told the exact way that *they* tested aids. What do we have to do so that the aids we get don't look so bad on our tests?

DR. CAUSEY: Our rejection rate is 8%; about one of every 12 aids we get does not live up to the curves we initially got. We have a rather large tolerance, but 8% are still rejected.

DR. ZELNICK (Hearing aid dealer): What is your tolerance limit?

DR. CAUSEY: I don't know at the moment, but it certainly exceeds ±2 dB.

DR. HARRIS: The hearing aid industry is, at the moment, formulating some final statements on how to test these items.

V. A. STANDARDS

DR. CAUSEY: The Food and Drug Administration has established performance standards. The V. A. standards will probably be tighter. We look at three samples of each model and average the frequency response of all three to develop the center line, so to speak, and then develop a tolerance around that.

CURRENT DEVELOPMENTS IN AURAL HABILITATION AND DISPENSING

Edward J. Hardick

Most of the energy in recent years has been expended in the refinement of diagnostic procedures, the development of new procedures for evaluating the subtle aspects of malfunction of the auditory system, the development of new training programs, and the establishment of audiology as a respected profession working primarily with the medical and educational commmunities. This is not to imply that audiologists have not contributed to the habilitation of individual hearing-impaired persons, but the same commitment of time, energy, and resources has not been devoted to the development of this aspect of audiological management. This has probably been a very normal evolutionary process with those problems most readily yielding to scientific inquiry being accomplished first.

UNMET NEED: AURAL REHABILITATION SERVICES

There have been problems in delivering aural habilitation services because of the difficulty in providing them before the sale of the hearing aid and the equally great difficulty in securing the return of these people after the sale. An increasing number of audiologists have become aware that the tremendous strides made by audiology and the medical sciences over the years have not significantly altered the need for habilitative programs or the need for audiologists, and their colleagues in related disciplines, to push back the frontiers in this area. Children are still born with profound hearing losses, while other children develop postnatal sensorineural hearing losses. Our noisy industrial society increases the number of hearing-impaired adults, and an increasing lifespan produces greater numbers of elderly people with auditory impairments. The literature is replete with studies demonstrating that: (1) many children wearing hearing aids do not develop auditory skills to their maximum, (2) from 50–80% of the hearing aids worn by children are defective, deficient, or inappropriate, (3) parents have very poor understanding of the care and function of their child's hearing and hearing aid, (4) too many elderly patients have hearing aids that are not useful to them, or at least not useful without other services, and (5) amplification is not used maximally in oral or total communication educational settings.

Despite technological advances in the hearing aid industry, the benefits of amplification still fall far short because realistic habilitative goals are not accomplished. It is apparent that there are serious shortcomings in the delivery of all services to the hearing impaired from birth to old age. These are most apparent at the ends of the age continuum. It is imperative that audiology take more of a leadership role in the delivery of services aimed at improving the communication performance of all hearing-impaired people.

NEW ROLES FOR AUDIOLOGISTS

Many audiologists have been aware of the shortcomings in the delivery of habilitative services. Three areas have emerged that require change or development.

Educational Audiology

Audiologists must expand their involvement with hearing-impaired children and with teachers of the hearing impaired. In order to accomplish these two goals, new ways must be sought to improve the quality and quantity of services offered in established clinical programs. More importantly, audiological services should be available on a continuing basis to *all* hearing-impaired children in an educational setting.

Hearing Aid Dispensing

The traditional hearing aid dispensing system is a severe deterrent to the delivery of high quality habilitative services at all age levels. Change in this traditional system is mandatory not only because of abuses that have forced legislatures to license hearing aid dealers as a means of regulating business practices, but also because consumer groups have again and again documented the inadequacy of these laws to protect the consumer. This system, as it presently exists, inserts a discontinuity in professional service that prohibits the delivery of other aspects of the necessary monitoring and habilitative program. The after-purchase services that the hearing aid dealer provides either are not provided, are severely lacking in quality, are too random, or are totally irrelevant to the habilitative goals of the audiologist and the needs of the hearing impaired.

Research Areas

Research programs in all areas of the habilitative process are needed. This includes the development of new tests, materials, and clinical procedures for evaluating the communication deficit of the hearing impaired diagnostically. These tests, which could provide a means for defining a sensory deficit in operational terms, would be the basis for determining optimal amplification which, in most cases, is the cornerstone of a successful habilitation program.

ACADEMY OF REHABILITATIVE AUDIOLOGY

As a charter member of the Academy of Rehabilitative Audiology, which was founded in 1966, as Editor of the "Journal of the Academy of Rehabilitative Audiology," and as President of this organization in 1975, I have witnessed the emergence of these three problem areas. The Academy of Rehabilitative Audiology was formed by a small group of audiologists who were concerned about the fact that insufficient attention was being directed toward the habilitation process in training programs, in research, and in clinical services. This group agreed that, although the profession had made significant strides in many directions, the status quo in habilitation had been maintained for too long. The Academy, through annual meetings and summer institutes, through the encouragement of program development and modification, and through the establishment of a journal, has significantly contributed to the following accomplishments:

Increased Awareness of Aural Rehabilitation Services

1. An increase in the number of sessions and papers presented on the topic of aural habilitation at the Annual Meeting of the American Speech and Hearing Association.
2. An increased concern on the part of employers for audiologists who are interested and knowledgeable in various aspects of the habilitative process.

3. An increased activity level of the American Speech and Hearing Association Committee on Aural Rehabilitation. The recent publication by Freeland et al., "The Audiologist: Responsibilities in the Habilitation of the Auditorily Handicapped" (1974) exemplifies this increasing awareness by audiologists of the necessity of changes in the delivery of service system.

4. The increased awareness that services to hearing-impaired children in the educational setting are in need of significant change. This has been highlighted by the report of the Joint Committee on Audiology and Education of the Deaf in its "Guidelines for Audiology Programs in Educational Settings for Hearing-Impaired Children" (1975).

5. The development of the "Journal of the Academy of Rehabilitative Audiology" has provided a forum for professionals who have something to say about aural habilitation. It also allows the Academy to disseminate the Proceedings of its Institutes and the deliberation of its committees. Anyone can be a contributor and anyone can be a subscriber.

Relationship between ARA and ASHA

1. An increased awareness by the American Speech and Hearing Association of the need for, and role of, special interest groups in the continued development of the profession.

2. In 1971 the Academy forwarded the following resolution to the American Speech and Hearing Association:

> "Be it resolved, that the participants in the Second Academy of Rehabilitative Audiology Institute urge the American Speech and Hearing Association to immediately address itself in the strongest possible terms to the issues of the audiologist and the dispensing of hearing aids."
> "Be it resolved, that the essential and crucial issue in the ethical dispensing of hearing aids is the quality of professional service in audiologic habilitation following, as well as preceding, the fitting and dispensing of the device rather than the economic aspects."

Educational Audiology

An increased awareness to better prepare audiologists for working with the hearing-impaired child in the educational setting. The academy has served as a forum for discussing this need, and the journal has recently published articles on educational and training models for a professional who has been termed an educational or school audiologist.

Task Forces on Aural Rehabilitation

From 1972 to 1975, the academy has devoted itself to the activities of the 14 task forces who addressed themselves to what were considered vital issues related to aural habilitation. Two of these task forces combined their efforts, invited in outside consultants, and have produced a report entitled, "Standards and Recommendations for Hearing Aids and Auditory Trainers." This report has been forwarded to various governmental agencies, to ANSI, and to the Hearing Aid Industry Conference. It presented a strong position on electroacoustical characteristics and the improvements and standardization of other aspects of hearing aid design and operation. The experience with these task forces made it clear that several issues needed increased attention, so the task force concept has been terminated. Five committees have been organized to address themselves to these issues: Amplification, Educational Models and Continuing Education, Research in Aural Habilitation, Aural Habilitation Programs and Services, and Hearing Aid Evaluation Procedures.

MODELS FOR DISPENSING HEARING AIDS

The most current issue today concerns the delivery of hearing aids to the hearing impaired. Several models are being advanced by professionals, hearing aid dealers, consumer groups, and federal agencies. Some of these are: dispensing without profit by audiologists, prescription, generic recommendations, and dispensing with profit by audiologists.

Some of these models have different meanings for different people depending upon the frame of reference from which they choose to view the issue. To some extent, these models may be looked upon differently by individuals from specific geographic regions because of the forces impinging upon them which are different from those forces in other parts of the country. As long as these differences in meaning exist, there are all kinds of opportunities for individuals to write articles that will be enthusiastically received by some element of the population.

Prescriptive Hearing Aid Models

Another difficulty in dealing with these models is that, in addition to the "state of the art" questions, there are strong interprofessional and political implications. For example, I do not like the word "prescription" relating to hearing aids, but I don't like it for reasons other than those discussed by Dr. Harris in his recent publication in "Hearing Instruments" (1975). If "prescription" can be defined as ordering a specific name-brand agent for a condition, then I can write a hearing aid prescription for a substantial number of hearing-impaired patients. When a physician prescribes he may be choosing one of several medications that will serve the purpose. There is not always a presumption that it will cure or that it can be tolerated. That's not unlike what happens with hearing aids.

PROS AND CONS ON HEARING AID DISPENSING

The present hearing aid delivery system does not meet the needs of most hearing-impaired people. The fact that audiologists can now ethically dispense hearing aids is a step forward in providing comprehensive habilitative services and giving the consumer some choice. This seems like a wise course of action for audiologists who feel frustrated in their attempts to deliver comprehensive services. Consumer groups, however, have a tendency to be opposed to the dispensing of hearing aids by audiologists because of the inherent possibility of conflict of interest. It is a legitimate and understandable concern based on the results of documented abuses by other professions who diagnose as well as treat. It is natural, then, for consumer groups to urge separation of the prescriber from the salesperson. I have no difficulty with this concept, providing the function of the seller is limited to providing the device and the necessary maintenance and service to keep it functioning—while all other pre- and postsale services are rendered by professionals, preferably audiologists. This would necessitate the direct involvement of the audiologist in habilitative procedures and the development of relevant research that will hopefully speed up the process from "art form" to "science." Audiologists should keep themselves informed of all the issues and the effects they will have on the welfare of the hearing impaired.

"GENERIC" RECOMMENDATIONS OF HEARING AIDS

During the present Michigan legislative session (1975–76) hearing aid dealers are pushing for law changes that would require audiologists to recommend hearing aids on a generic basis. Audiologists might be prepared for similar action in other states. The following is part of a letter written by the author to a Michigan legislator on the topic of generic recommendations:

> Hearing aid evaluations normally consist of the selection of a number of hearing aids from various manufacturers that generally might be considered to be from the same "generic" family, placing these hearing aids on the patient and objectively determining speech discrimination performance. Usually when a specific hearing aid is recommended for an individual, it is based upon the fact that the hearing aid has yielded the highest understanding of speech. Sometimes a specific hearing aid is recommended even when all hearing aids yield the same results because the patient has expressed a subjective preference for that particular hearing aid. The patient may use a variety of criteria to make that decision including quality of sound, physical comfort, ease of operation of controls, cosmetic preferences, etc. Normally, hearing clinics that recommend specific hearing aids do not make capricious

recommendations. Most of the people who choose to come to an audiology clinic, rather than to a hearing aid dealer's office, are interested in the specific recommendation of one hearing aid to avoid the uncertainties of dealing in the marketplace with a vendor. When recommending a specific hearing aid, the audiologist does not pretend that the hearing aid is the only one in the universe that could be used by that individual. The audiologist does know that the hearing aid recommended performs as well as or better than a representative sample of hearing aids of similar performance characteristics. The audiologist is not going to evaluate each conceivable hearing aid that might provide benefit to the patient, but, by the same token, neither is the hearing aid dealer.

COMPETENCY OF HEARING AID DEALERS

People accept the fact that hearing aid dealers are not qualified by virtue of training, experience, or instrumentation for performing diagnostic hearing tests. This has been demonstrated in various studies reported by consumer groups. The hearing aid dealer is no better qualified to perform tests involving the selection of hearing aids than he is to perform diagnostic testing. Most hearing aid dealers in the state of Michigan do not have the necessary instrumentation for measuring benefit from hearing aids. Furthermore, most do not have the necessary electroacoustic equipment to measure the performance characteristics of hearing aids.

In addition to the limitations of the hearing aid dealer in terms of expertise or instrumentation to fill a generic prescription, there is a major problem with the use of the term "generic" relative to hearing aids. Most people are accustomed to thinking about the word "generic" as it applies to the prescription of chemical products. Unfortunately, the same principles may not be as easily applied to physics. Not all parameters of hearing aid performance are measured, partly out of industry reluctance and partly because there are no well-accepted tests for some of the parameters. If the parameters of hearing aid performance (gain, maximum output, and frequency response) were employed as the operational definition of generic, and I certainly hope that this would not be the case, there still would be substantial differences between hearing aids in any pool of generically "equivalent" hearing aids. Some of the hearing aids might have a tone control, a telephone coil, a front-facing microphone, or a top or rear-mounted microphone. Some aids employ peak clipping, while others use various forms of automatic volume control. Some have directional microphones, varying amounts of harmonic and transient distortion, and the taper of the volume control may be significantly different. In the broadest sense of the term, these hearing aids would not be generic equivalents. This would be like prescribing aspirin, knowing that it contained additional ingredients that were unknown in amount and effect. For many patients, all of these are important parameters that affect the benefit provided, and not to take them into account when recommending an aid would be indefensible.

It is hoped that these comments will provide some impetus for further discussion of current developments in aural habilitation and dispensing.

LITERATURE CITED

Freeland, E. E., M. J. Hill, J. Jeffers, N. D. Matkin, R. W. Stream, H. Tobin, and M. R. Costello. 1974. The audiologist: Responsibilities in the habilitation of the auditorily handicapped. Asha 16: 68–70.
Harris, J. D. 1975. Prescription hearing aids. Hearing Instruments 26(2): 11–12.
Report of the Joint Committee on Audiology and Education of the Deaf. 1975. Guidelines for Audiology Programs in Educational Settings for Hearing Impaired Children. Asha 17: 17–20.

DISCUSSION

CONFLICT OF INTEREST IN HEARING AID DISPENSING

AUDIENCE MEMBER: The conflict of interest in dispensing hearing aids was discussed. Do you have any observations on the realities of that matter?

DR. HARDICK: People who go into audiology have a strong puritan ethic. Over the last 10 years, many audiologists have wrestled with that. Those audiologists who realized the importance of total interaction with their clients came to the conclusion that they had to become involved with hearing aids in one way or another and all rehabilitative aspects of whatever particular patient they were working with, whether that meant dispensing aids themselves or ordering through a salesperson and then following up themselves. What hasn't happened is that audiologists haven't gotten together to talk about this issue until recently. Certainly, a conflict of interest exists in all professions. Why audiologists get so hung up on it, I don't know. Unfortunately, at the moment, audiologists are coming to a crossroad requiring a change in how they do things, while, at the same time, the consumer has awakened to the fact that *he* perhaps ought to be interested in the things that happen to him.

CONSUMER OPPOSITION TO DISPENSING BY AUDIOLOGISTS

I've been involved in Michigan in legislation in the past 5 years and developed a liaison with consumer groups. I see it quite dramatically: when I talk to them about audiologists dispensing hearing aids, a look of horror crosses their faces. They are adamantly opposed to it, their philosophy being that if it is possible to set apart the prescriber from the prescribee, one ought to do it. That's unfortunate. Most of these consumer groups do not know much about hearing aids or hearing impairment. They tend to approach all problems from this point of view. It's not an impossible situation, but it does complicate things. In addition to convincing one's colleagues of the importance of the issue, audiologists need to talk to larger groups of people. I don't view dispensing as a problem.

PROPOSED FDA REGULATIONS: PRESCRIPTIVE HEARING AIDS

AUDIENCE MEMBER: Would you give an educated guess about what statements will be made by the Food and Drug Administration and Department of Health, Education, and Welfare regarding hearing aids?

DR. HARDICK: My information from Washington is that if the Food and Drug Administration defines an aid as a health prosthetic device then it almost automatically becomes a prescriptive item.

DR. ZELNICK (Hearing aid dealer): What is your definition of "prescriptive item"? This is the big question mark. Does it mean medical clearance or a more definitive prescription of a type of hearing aid? It is universally accepted that medical clearance is required. The next step is: will prescription be required *as well as* medical clearance? By medical clearance, I mean the otologist writing a prescription that a hearing aid is required in a particular case: it does *not* mean the exact definition as to model or make or performance characteristics of a particular aid. This is where some of the controversy sets in. How far do you go in your definition of a prescriptive device?

DR. HARDICK: That is really an open question. I said "prescription." Obviously the Food and Drug Administration and the Health, Education, and Welfare (HEW) task force is going to be under pressure from various special interest groups to have certain things happen. The National Hearing Aid Society (NHAS), for example, has just agreed to medical clearance for all hearing-impaired people. So NHAS has its orientation to the problem; the American Speech and Hearing Association (ASHA) has its input. The original HEW task force called for prescription by otolaryngologists or audiologists which would be similar to the prescription of glasses by ophthalmologists or optometrists. ASHA is backing that, although they are perhaps unhappy with the word "prescription" because of its possible connotation, and probably encouraging the possibility of audiologists "prescribing" in any fashion they think to be in the best interest of the hearing-impaired person. That would mean a specific brand if that seemed to be appropriate, or generic or multiple brands. That's a presumption on my part. Consumer groups have input, the Nader groups, grey panthers, pushing for prescriptions without necessarily dealing with the nitty-gritty of what that entails. Audiologists should become as familiar with these issues as possible.

DR. HARRIS: Dr. Causey, you're on the ground in Washington—what are your comments?

ASHA POSITION ON HEARING AIDS

DR. CAUSEY: If the women in the audience will forgive me for almost a sexist remark, I have a mental picture of ASHA as an old woman who lifts her skirts, so as not to get them muddy, as, in the background, a tidal wave of gigantic proportions tumbles and rumbles toward her. ASHA has been concerned about small points, when in reality something big is happening that they are not yet attuned to. The question is national health care and it is just around the corner. A national health care bill on hearing aids is not going to be passed until a system is developed whereby aids are given to the public with: (1) the determination as to who gets one made by an unbiased individual, and (2) low cost. Otherwise, the taxpayers could not afford it.

It behooves every audiologist to become involved somehow with hearing aids in a meaningful fashion. This will be determined by geographical location, state laws, relationship with area dealers, the kind of rapport established, and the distribution system at the moment. Every audiologist owes it to himself, to the hearing impaired, and to his profession to become fully involved with hearing aids as a rehabilitative tool. I would say, "Do not let anything ASHA says or intimates stop you from being so involved."

DR. HARRIS: You realize this is being taped, Dr. Causey? On another occasion, I was asked if I minded if my remarks were taped. I responded that I didn't see any reason why they shouldn't be. When I got the tape, it was pretty noisy, but when I took it back to the lab to try to clean it up with the Dolby noise suppression technique, it turned out that the hiss was coming not from the tape but from the audience.

AUDIENCE MEMBER: Do we know how many audiologists are actually dispensing hearing aids?

DR. HARDICK: It's a relatively large number, probably in excess of 100.

REFERRALS TO AUDIOLOGIST DISPENSERS

AUDIENCE MEMBER: I am an audiologist dispensing hearing aids in private practice. One of my biggest problems is to get other professionals to refer their patients to me. What would you do to remedy that?

DR. CAUSEY: Why do you think referrals are not made?

AUDIENCE MEMBER: One of the reasons is that they have already established good relationships with people with whom they have been working. Also, audiologists still think that hearing aids are untouchable things for audiologists. We have to support our own people in this field.

DR. CAUSEY: Are the hearing aids that you dispense sold at your cost?

AUDIENCE MEMBER: Yes.

DR. CAUSEY: If you charge a fee for services, isn't the total package then costing the patient less than the other route?

AUDIENCE MEMBER: Yes. Some people feel that the so-called master plan has a low price, but clients don't get some of the services that my office provides.

AUDIENCE MEMBER: I live in Westchester, in Yonkers, where I propose to open a private practice. In Yonkers, with a population of 214,000, there are five Ear, Nose, and Throat (ENT) men, six hearing aid dealers, three ENT clinics and hospitals with a fourth very close. In that metropolitan area where there is no shortage of professionals, there is only one audiologist, working three mornings a week in one of the hospitals. I sent out just a brief letter saying that I was thinking of opening a private practice in audiology and describing my services. I sent it out to all the ENT doctors and all the other kinds of doctors. I met up against an absolute stone wall from the ENT men. One doctor had a dealer who bounced into his office every 2 months with the latest thing and a big sales pitch. Another physician said, "Of course you can make fitting hearing aids as difficult as you want. If you want me to send my patients to you, you have to tell me what you would do that the dealers don't." These physicians don't hire audiologists. They have nurses.

AUDIENCE MEMBER: The persons responsible, even in Connecticut, are the doctors. They do the hiring, set up the budget, do the referring, and they also set up the programs. There is little knowledge or appreciation of the audiologist.

PROFIT MOTIVE IN DISPENSING

DR. DOERFLER: I am somewhat confused about what appear to be some inconsistencies. Dr. Hardick indicated that the concern of the audiologists should be the quality of the service and not control through economics. This young lady was talking about being shunned by her colleagues because she lost her audiological virginity. When Dr. Causey responded to her, his question was: "Are you selling for profit or are you arranging your economics so that the money comes through a roundabout way through service?" This kind of approach bothers me. It is clearly antagonistic to the statement that Dr. Hardick made and becomes a dictation of the way in which audiologists have to jimmy their economics to fit a pattern that somehow makes them acceptable, whereas if they did it another way, with the same quality of service, they aren't acceptable.

DR. CAUSEY: I was trying to offer her a way in which to bring about referrals by pointing out to the fellow audiologists that, for about the same cost their patients are buying directly from dealers, she can offer the professional evaluation and the hearing aid without adding these costs on to the dealer. I was trying to give her something to point to in order to bring in referrals.

DR. DOERFLER: The question that should be asked by fellow audiologists is, "What is the quality of service that she is giving?"—not this kind of economic financial wizardry that somehow changes the way things are done.

DR. ZELNICK (Hearing aid dealer): As a hearing aid dispenser for over 26 years, and as an audiologist with the doctorate in hearing science, I can see both sides of the picture. I advocate commercial audiology, and the prime consideration, as Dr. Doerfler so aptly states, is not so much the cost or economics involved as it is the quality of service offered by the dispenser. This is what the otologist is concerned about in making a referral. He is concerned not only with the quality of service, but also with reliability. Will that person be there to perform this type of service 6 months, 1 year, 5 years later? These relationships are not built up overnight. It takes many years to develop and build good images and to build dependency so that the professional community involved in making referals will have the confidence to refer to a particular agency, whether audiologist or dispenser.

Finally, hearing aid dispensing with competence and efficiency is a tremendous financial investment. Well-established hearing aid offices around the country have a large investment in all kinds of equipment in order to test aids properly and to set up proper servicing facilities in their particular institutions or commercial facilities.

DOOR-TO-DOOR HEARING AID SALES

DR. GERSTMAN: Primarily we are facing what every pioneer faces: doing something controversial and new. Therefore, before they change, people who have done things one way will want to see if this is a better way. My experience has been that the success ratio becomes very high after you break through that first couple of months and the professional community realizes that you are not going to sell door-to-door. There is a professional office versus a commercial one. It's not just "so-and-so's hearing center" emphasizing the aid and not emphasizing rehabilitation services. I would just give some comfort and enthusiasm to you both because people across the country have shown it can work. I know of 47 audiologists in private practice across the country and 112 facilities. Even though I disagree with some of the statements made here, the system in the past of selling hearing aids door-to-door is not going to be very successful.

ROLE OF THE AUDIOLOGIST

AUDIENCE MEMBER: Certain issues seem to be recurring. The problems that were expressed by this woman lead to several assumptions. It is not the responsibility of other professions to find out what audiologists do. Audiologists have the responsibility to clarify exactly what they do. The fact that an otologist who happens to be working with me in a particular area does not really know what audiologists do raises a question: what do audiologists do that is different from a hearing aid dealer? This is a legitimate question, and must be responded to seriously. Audiologists cannot blame anyone except themselves. It is their responsibility basically on all levels to clarify the nature of the services that they provide. In private practice there are several approaches which can be taken. The obvious approach, which is probably going to receive some negative response, is the one this young lady described. You simply can't call up people and say, "Hey, I'm here. I have a service and I would like referrals." It seems not the way to go about it. It is also a naive assumption that otologists and residents in large medical centers know what audiologists do.

AUDIENCE MEMBER: Dr. Gerstman has some input to the resident program in the Boston area. Is it true that total time devoted to audiology in a 3-year program is 1 week?

DR. GERSTMAN: No, it's more than that—but still it is not enough.

COST ACCOUNTING FOR HEARING AID DISPENSING

AUDIENCE MEMBER: How do audiologists cope with costs and the reluctance of their own administration to meet them?

DR. DOERFLER: The first step would be to take a very hard look at their own expenses and be able to justify them. This is a step often skipped. I wish I had a dollar for every letter I get from clinics and administrators of hospital rehabilitation centers who write to me every year and say, "We're starting a clinic," or "We want to revise our fee schedule. Would you send us a copy of yours?" It's unbelievable that no one knows what their costs are! Until audiologists can really specify their costs, they are not going to be able to sell a service to a third party.

RESEARCH NEEDS

AUDIENCE MEMBER: There is now a federal regulation requiring that all children be tested for hearing. In checking through New York state, there are few communities that have the facilities to do this preschool hearing testing. In Westchester, when a proposal was made, the local government would not provide funds ($53,000) to improve the acoustical standards of the place where the children were being tested.

DR. HARDICK: Funding of that kind of research has always been a significant problem, which goes along with my comments about the diagnostic aspects of audiology holding sway for years because they are very dramatic. Perhaps the HEW task force will change that since they are talking about funding this kind of research.

DEVELOPMENT OF A TEST INSTRUMENT FOR SPEECH DISCRIMINATION

Hubert L. Gerstman

This report summarizes the major aspects of work completed to date in the development of a new sentence test for speech discrimination.

The object of this investigation is the creation of a test instrument that may be used as part of a standard battery in defining an individual's auditory discrimination abilities. It is recognized that a realistic statement of such abilities, for clinical purposes, should measure not only the peripheral hearing system but also the patient's cognitive potential. Therefore, this investigation sought to control for effects of familiarity of words and levels of semantic predictability, so that sentences requiring various degrees of cognitive ability on the part of the listener could be generated as test items.

INITIAL DESIGN OF SENTENCE MATERIALS

In order to effect such controls, standardized procedures for producing sentences were created. In simplifying the problems of obtaining responses from listeners and of scoring responses, the sentences were designed to contain target words in final position. Monosyllabic nouns were used as

This project was supported by NINCDS, U.S. Department of Health, Education, and Welfare, contract 1-NS-4-2322.

these key words because they form a homogeneous set that can be more easily placed in a sentence context and they are more easily manipulated with respect to semantic properties in sentences. In order to maintain a reasonable degree of homogeneity with respect to word familiarity, words were selected to lie between approximately two and 150 occurrences per million, according to the Thorndike-Lorge count. For purposes of initial experimentation, 479 such monosyllabic nouns were selected.

Sentences in which the key words have four levels of predictability were developed:

Zero Predictability (PO)

This context is found in the presentation of standard, phonetically balanced word lists such as: "Say the word. . ." or "The next word is. . ." or (as in this study) "I will now say the word. . . ."

Low Predictability (PL)

These sentences are from five to eight syllables in length (the same limits apply to moderate predictability and high predictability sentences below) and can take virtually any noun, concrete or abstract in final position. Several hundred unique frames were generated, of seven different types. These contained contexts such as "talk about the. . . ," "call about the . . . ," or "problem with the. . . ." No two phrases were completely identical, although some might vary only in terms of the subject nouns.

Moderate Predictability (PM)

The generation rules here allowed the sentence to either be declarative or a question, but not of the "yes" or "no" type. Whereas in the PL situation, there were no "pointer" words in the context, so that virtually any noun could fit as the key word, in the PM situation there was one "pointer" feature preceding the key word, so that in a sentence like, "He walked on the. . . ," words such as "sky" would obviously be eliminated from consideration, while other words such as "road" would be considered more likely. PM sentences were generated for 95 of the key words.

High Predictability (PH)

The generation rules include the provision that each sentence should have at least two pointer features in the context. This would heavily load the concept and increase the probability of a correct response. Additional constraints were employed so that the key word would always receive the main stress. This eliminated the use of the target word in a compound. Thus a word like "cone" could not be used in the context of "ice cream cone" because of the unstressing of the last word occuring in this phrase. A total of 574 different PH sentences was generated according to these rules. For 95 of the nouns, two rival PH sentences were generated.

Examples of words with their associated sentence P levels follow:

Word = "germs."
>   PO = I will now say the word "germs."
>   PL = She should not have discussed the germs (no pointers).
>   PH = *Hospitals* should be *free* of germs (2 pointers).

Word = "clock."
>   PO = I will now say the word "clock."
>   PM = Would you please look at the clock? (1 pointer).
>   PH = We *heard* the *ticking* of the clock (2 pointers).

EXPERIMENTS DESIGNED TO EVALUATE MATERIALS

Two types of experiments were performed to evaluate the sentence materials and to provide an initial basis for the ultimate selection of items for a clinical test instrument. These experiments consisted of a set of paper-and-pencil tests to assess the predictability of key words in the PH sentences and a series of listening tests in which the intelligibility of the words in the various sentence types was determined when the sentences were presented in a background babble at several signal-to-babble ratios.

Assessing Predictability by Written Tests

These studies were carried out in a paper-and-pencil format with two groups of subjects. The purpose of this work was to provide some baseline information on the predictability of the key words for each PH item. These data comprise an independent, nonacoustic measurement of one aspect of the PH sentences. The output of these written experiments was a predictability score for each of the 574 PH sentences. The operational definition of predictability is the proportion of subjects who are able to supply the intended final word when a sentence is presented in written form without that word. We are not measuring the predictability of the entire sentence but only of its strength in pointing toward its last or key word. It should be noted that the number of pointer cues will be smaller in the acoustic experimentation as a result of signal-to-babble interference which we will discuss below.

The first group for the written experimentation consisted of 12 high school students with a mean age of 16. This was a prompted predictability experiment in that the vowel nucleus in the target word was indicated to the subject. His task was to write down the most likely monosyllabic target word that contained the given vowel. The prompt indicating of the vowel was introduced as a means of bringing the questionnaire situation into closer agreement with the acoustic presentation to be employed in the clinic.

The second group of high school students, with a mean age of 17, completed answer sheets similar to those above, but without the prompt. Figure 1 shows the results of these two independent experiments. These histograms demonstrate the face validity of the generation rules for the PH conditions and indicate that, even in the unprompted situation, the semantic predictability of the sentence contexts is high in most cases.

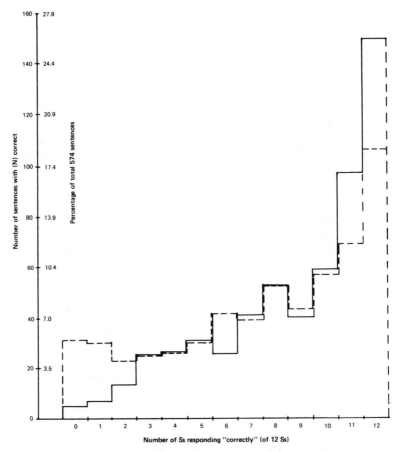

Figure 1. Summary of predictability experiments. *Dashed line*, performance of 12 Ss in the unprompted situation. *Solid line*, prompted.

The selection of items for the ultimate test instrument will utilize these data as a basis for eliminating sentences with low predictability.

Evaluation of Intelligibility of Materials

This experiment was planned to answer several questions within one overall design. These data will be used as a basis for specification of the first clinical version of the test instrument.

Experimental Hypotheses

Questions this experiment was designed to answer include:

1. What are the intelligibility functions? (Intelligibility versus signal-to-babble ratio for each target word in PH, PM, PL, and PO context.)
2. What is the effect of changes in the overall sound pressure level at which the babble is presented?
3. What are the relationships between paper-and-pencil predictability and the acoustic performance of a given sentence written according to generation rules which supposedly maximize predictability?
4. Are the PH sentences reliably different from the PL sentences for the same target words?
5. Is there any difference between the performance of PL and PO sentences for the same target words?
6. What kind of performance is exhibited by the sentences generated according to the PM rules?
7. Is the intelligibility function of the typical PM sentence different in *level* or *shape* from those of the PH or PL sentences?
8. Is the PM type of sentence a candidate for use in the ultimate test instrument?

Materials

The sentences were recorded in lists of 41 items each by a trained male talker. The masking stimulus was a babble of six different talkers (three men and three women) reading connected text, with each talker repeated twice, a total of 12 voices speaking simultaneously. The level of each of the individual voice contributions to the sound pressure level of the babble was balanced. The resulting signal is quite unintelligible and rather aversive.

Subjects

A total of 81 college-age subjects served in this experiment following several groups of pilot subjects whose data were used for adjustment of the stimulating conditions. All were screened for normal hearing. The 81 subjects whose data comprised the experimental results were run in 14 groups of from five to seven per group. Each subject heard a different set of 41 sentences in each of 14 different experimental conditions. Each subject listened to 1,722 test items. Within each list of 41 sentences, the items were either: (1) all PH sentences, (2) all PO sentences, or (3) mixed PM and PL sentences. The same target word occurred only once in a given list.

Test Procedures

Listening conditions were as follows: for most tests, the overall babble sound pressure level (BSPL) was set at 70 dB re 0.0002 dyne/cm^2, with five sound:babble ratios represented for the PH (PM = PL materials) and two for the PO materials. PH sentences were also tested at two sound:babble ratios at a higher babble level (85 dB BSPL). A Graeco-Latin square design was used to counterbalance the order of occurrence of these events. The subjects were run in the anechoic chamber of the Los Angeles facilities of Bolt, Beranek, and Newman. Subjects wore standard calibrated earphones, only one of which was excited by the signal. The nonpreferred ear was covered by the inactive transducer. A fixed, 7-second ISI was used. Subjects wrote their answers.

Results

Figure 2 shows a series of intelligibility functions, with the percentage correct on the ordinate and signal:babble ratio on the abscissa. Across all items the PH functions are steeper and more predictably accurate. PL functions typically lie to the right of PH, are more gradually sloping, and, most critically, essentially follow the PO data points. Thus, it is possible to conclude that the PL context may provide essentially the same information as the more traditional PB contexts (use of carrier phrases) while being more useful by being more directly comparable to the PH context. It is likely, therefore, that the final versions of this test will not include PO material.

Figure 3 compares the PL, PM, and PH sentences. If PL sentences fall substantially and consistently to the right of PH, it would be expected that sentences of moderate predictability would generate articulation functions that would lie between PH and PL curves. This is found to be the case, thus validating the generation rules for PM sentences. By the same token, one can probably discount their usefulness in that the PM sentences lie on a continuum of intelligibility and provide less leverage in the measurement of the contributions of context. We gain greater precision and minimize

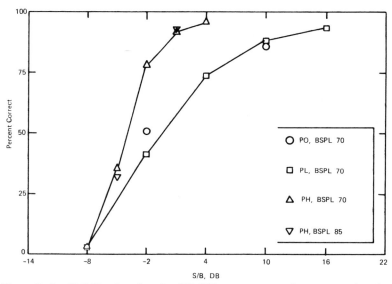

Figure 2. Intelligibility functions for 479 different target words as presented at three different context levels and at two babble SPL's. The insert associates context and babble level with the plotted symbols.

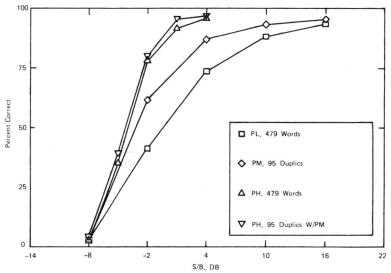

Figure 3. Comparison between key-word intelligibility functions generated by PH, PM, and PL context levels. The two PH curves are generated by different numbers of sentences: 479 for the base-down triangles, 95 for the apex-down triangles. The PL and PM functions are derived from the same numbers of sentences, respectively.

the effects of measurement error by maximizing the contextural differences (i.e., using PL and PH sentences), while retaining all other controls,
such as similarity in rhythmic pattern in PL and PH sentences. It is likely,
then, that the final versions of the test instrument will consist only of PL
and PH sentences. Figure 3 also shows that the 95 words that were
duplicated in different PH sentences have essentially the same function as
that based on the full set of words.

TOWARD DESIGN OF THE TEST INSTRUMENT

It is our intention to make a preliminary selection of items for a test
instrument based on results obtained up to the present and to carry out
some evaluation of the instrument with a clinical population. Item selection will be based on some, or all, of the following considerations. The
objective will be to produce a subset of items and eventually a series of
equivalent similar subsets whose PH and PL functions will be even more
separated that they are at present. This will occur primarily through the
rejection of items that do not contribute to the desired separation between
these curves, subject to the constraint that reasonable phonetic balance is
maintained among the items in a test. We shall aim toward subsets
containing 50 items, although it is possible that we will find that 50-item
presentations may be too many for clinic use, thereby allowing us to enjoy
a shorter list, with good statistical assurance, while increasing the number
of available equivalent lists themselves.

The final version of the test instrument has not been dictated by
activities to date. It is likely that tape recordings will be generated in
several different formats for use by the clinician and/or researcher. There
are a number of choices available to us at this point: (1) sentences with
key words imbedded in a variety of signal/babble conditions; (2) sentences
in tracks separated from the babble—to be mixed by the clinician.

Procedural considerations are furthermore dependent on experimental
results pertaining to the maximum of articulation curves (PL versus PH).
The manner of training and the approach to level setting remain to be
determined. Options include: (1) tracking signal/babble to a percentage
score criterion; (2) specific sensation level (SL); and (3) use of fixed
babble sound pressure level (BSPL).

DISCUSSION

This material is presented because the objectives of NINCDS were to
create a sentence-discrimination test that would be useful for work with
the hearing impaired and particularly for purposes of hearing aid evalua-

tion. In seeking a more realistic and natural test which includes evaluation of cognitive skills as well as aspects of the peripheral mechanism, the difficulties in attempting to measure such items as "central factors" have been considered. The test is, therefore, being designed to control for such factors. A patient not able to score well under PH conditions definitely needs other assistance than that provided by amplification only. On the other hand, a patient scoring very well under PL conditions, who has been identified as one with a peripheral handicap, is an excellent hearing aid candidate who does not even need maximum cues for identification of speech stimuli. It is expected that patients whose performance deviates from the norms generated by the current investigations will have demonstrated their atypical listening and "coping" skills and will, therefore, benefit from more precise counseling by the clinical audiologist. The intention is to generate norms relative to the PL/PH *difference* scores which are expected to generate clinical utility in a "single" number or classification. Future investigators may then be able to correlate these different scores with states of auditory efficiency or pathology.

EXPECTED VALUES

It is expected that those of us engaged in basic clinical and normative data gathering will benefit from the creation of a well-defined and validated test instrument. Beyond those investigations dealing with the hearing aid user, it is expected that this test instrument may become useful in the diagnostic battery and that investigations will be forthcoming that demonstrate how a variety of specific diagnostic categories perform in the use of this test. It is hoped that this test will show greater differentiation between defined diagnostic groups and that specific percentage losses will be found for such pathologies as: conductive, cochlear, retrocochlear or pathway lesions, and cortical lesions.

Such descriptive categories may be defined in much the same way as, for instance, Jerger has defined these diagnostic groups on other popularly used tests.

It is hoped that this test instrument will provide the clinician with a new and sensitive discrimination test that exercises some control over cognitive variables and that may serve a useful purpose in hearing aid evaluation procedures.

ACKNOWLEDGMENTS

The project acknowledges the work of its team members: in experimental design and analysis, A. W. F. Huggins, Barbara Freeman, Jeffrey Berliner,

Walter Hawkins; in preparation and execution of the acoustic experiments, Karl Pearsons, Sanford Fidell, Sam Tamooka, Brian Curtis; for overall guidance, Ray Nickerson; and for consultation services, Hubert L. Gerstman of New England Medical Center Hospital and Rhoda Morrison and Harold F. Schuknecht of Massachusetts Eye and Ear Infirmary.

Co-principal investigators were Daniel N. Kalikow and Kenneth N. Stevens of Bolt, Beranek, and Newman, Inc., 50 Moulton Street, Cambridge, Massachusetts.

SUMMARY

J. Donald Harris

THE V. A. AS A MODEL AUDIOLOGY CLINIC

Although Veterans Administration audiology clients hardly typify those of the usual clinic, being adult males with trauma and presbycusis the overwhelming diagnosis, the V. A. program is often looked to as a guide since Ken Johnson and Bernard Anderman first set it up. The program was able to attract scores of doctorate level audiologists. It had the full use of the excellent staff at the Bureau of Standards to design and run physical tests on samples of every aid submitted and it solicited a very active consultant group under the direction of Professor Raymond Carhart, the pioneer and still certainly the foremost authority in the field.

Could not the whole country follow the lead of the V. A.? Although the tendency in any large organization is to freeze practice, the V. A. has continued to be innovative. Most of all, it has deliberately resisted the plan of promulgating specifications for aids it will put on contract. This would have the consequence that companies would manufacture for the V. A. bidding a "V. A.-aid" which might have little relation to the product they would distribute to their usual dispensing outlets. Thus, the V. A. has the opportunity to pick and choose among all the models an inventive industry can contrive. Second, the V. A. has filled its top positions with research-trained individuals who themselves conduct first-rate work and use their positions of leverage to create conditions conducive to research for staff members. One V. A. center, for example, gave a leave of absence, at half pay, to a young man to come to our lab and do his dissertation with the Zwislocki impedance bridge, and another recent Ph.D. was given $4,000 worth of new equipment and released time to do some in-house research. The V. A. is moving toward setting up in-house centers for audiological research in hearing aids.

NEED FOR RESEARCHERS

A modern industry would quickly die if it did not spend a far greater percentage on basic research than the profession of audiology now devotes to its clinical research. The lifeblood of the profession has been pumped into it year after year by those devoted clinical researchers such as Carhart, Lassman, Bergman, Bangs, Hardy, Jerger, and Doerfler. Unless some of their students continue in research, the profession will stagnate and many unsolved problems will be preempted by other groups.

COMMENTS ON DR. CAUSEY'S PRESENTATION

In this regard, we could all take lessons from both the breadth and the depth of view which Dr. Causey brings to the problems of amplification in his population. While statistics show that the V. A. usually lags somewhat behind hearing aid dispensers (it was slower, for example, in accepting ear-level aids with gains of over 40 dB and in accepting eyeglass aids), a bit of inertia is not necessarily bad. Newer aids, with more cosmetic appeal, are often acoustically inferior to older models. Enough flexibility is now built into the V. A. system that changes are made for the better all the time. Dr. Causey's view is apt—that of traditional audiology as an old woman raising her long skirts to avoid getting wet by little waves at water's edge, while a tsunami 30 feet high is racing to shore. Everything about the hearing aid and its uses has been in constant change for decades, and the rate of change will only accelerate. In another decade our current prostheses and practices will seem at best droll and at worst aboriginal.

COMMENTS ON DR. HARDICK'S PRESENTATION

Dr. Hardick has presented strong reasons for the audiologist to dispense aids, and I agree with him. Obviously, adults with certain types and degrees of hypacusis can stroll into a hearing aid salesman's office, receive any of many good aids, and need nothing further. But few hypacusics have problems so simple. A newborn patient may need an internist, a general surgeon, a biochemist, a neurophysiologist, a medical audiologist, and a pediatrician to identify a sensory defect, establish etiology, and create a medical regimen. In his first years the patient may need a language expert to interact with the family to teach that family how to create speech and language in that child. He may need a pediatric audiologist to develop the use of auditory cues. He may need a person trained in the special problems of the deaf-blind or the quite different special problems of the hard-of-hearing mental retardate. Few audiologists could provide all these services, but, of all professions today, it is audiology within which those persons and training programs exist to diagnose the patient's real needs and mobilize the community's resources. The profession of hearing aid fitting must be woven so closely into the profession of audiology that, for many patients, the two must be one.

UPGRADING HEARING AID DEALER COMPETENCY

The thought is being widely expressed that every hearing aid dispenser should have training equivalent to that of an undergraduate major in audiology. This may sound utopian, but large steps have already been taken in this and other countries; it is an idea whose time has come. Two solutions are simultaneously possible: (1) to upgrade the competence of those now dispensing aids and (2) to attract into the work those who are already audiologically trained. To be fully qualified to work with all persons requires considerable training in audiological topics.

"But," one says, "why do you need to be able to design and carry out aural rehabilitation regimes when for many mature patients they are not needed?" I think here of an analogy: With a Zeiss scope, a micromanipulator, and a tiny drill I have created a parallel-sided hole in the bone near the round window and inserted a 0.005-inch insulated wire into the perilymph, but only in the cat, not in the human. With these tools I could scrape away some deposits and mobilize the stapes in an otosclerotic human. But I would be no better fitted to do this than a gorilla steering a car, having no notion of the complications I might see, of variations of the facial nerve, of cholesteotomas, of the tympanic plexus in that area of the human ear, of the course of the chorda tympani. My patient would have his stapes mobilized all right, but his tongue would have no taste, his face would sag on one side, and he would likely die of chagrin when he found Medicare would not pay for my services.

Just as only a trained otologist should attempt even what is now the most routine mobilization, it takes a knowledgeable and experienced hearing aid dispenser to achieve success, in the more difficult cases, in selecting and adapting what apparatus is currently available to the needs of the individual hypacusic. Only a trained audiologist, however, can understand and deal effectively with the total communication problems of a person for whom even the best-fitted aid is only one of perhaps many steps leading to full attainment of the human condition.

COMMENTS ON DR. GERSTMAN'S PAPER

Dr. Gerstman has given us a good look at the construction of a set of speech materials likely to be of great research value. There are hundreds of sentences for which precise information on predictability and intelligibility of key words will be at hand. It is a good bet that, when further processed, these will serve much better than the spondees and PB lists to sample the colloquial speech which the hypacusic must handle with its distortions, modulation, and noise. The profession needs taped versions of these sentences to use instead of current materials.

The further suggestion has merit that a clinically important sign might be the difference for a particular patient between an intelligibility score for sentences with high key-word predictability versus the score for sentences with low key-word predictability. The thought is that a person scoring relatively well under conditions of low predictability may be a good candidate for a hearing aid. This suggestion will undergo validation research in a number of clinics.

ELECTROACOUSTICAL STANDARDS

INTRODUCTION

Laura Ann Wilber

This panel was designed to provide insight into the procedures and practices of the measurement of hearing aids. We will not be concerned about the way an individual's performance with a hearing aid is measured, but only with the manner in which the electronic device itself can be defined acoustically.

PROMULGATION OF A NEW STANDARD

It is important to initially understand the concept of standards. In designing any standard for measurement one must first determine what has to be measured. Next one must decide whether the method of measurement must be specified. Related to that one must determine how much tolerance on the procedure for measurement may be accepted, and one must then decide whether the standard must require certain parameters to reach acceptance levels and what tolerances, if any, may be allowed on a measured characteristic. For example, when we talk about the measurement of gain of a hearing aid, it must first be determined if gain is to be measured. Then it must be decided whether gain must be measured at all frequencies or any combination thereof. Next it must be decided whether gain must be measured with the hearing aid turned full on or at some other setting and whether the input level to the hearing aid must be specified. If the input is to be specified, what level and what frequency or frequencies will be required? Finally, after one has decided *what* to measure and *how* to measure it, one must decide if one needs to set other types of standards. For example, should it be necessary to specify the maximum gain which a hearing aid can have or the minimum gain that the hearing aid could have? Then it must be decided how much tolerance will be allowed for a given instrument to say it still meets its own manufacturer's standards. For example, if the manufacturer says the maximum gain is 60 dB, would 62 or 82 dB be out of line?

HISTORY OF DEVELOPMENT OF STANDARDS

The measurement of hearing aids has been going on since hearing aids were first developed. It appears, however, that the first standard which was developed for the measurement of hearing aids in general was one created by the International Electrotechnical Commission (IEC) which developed its standard in 1959. The standard is IEC Publication 118 entitled "Recommended Methods for Measurements of the Electro-acoustical Characteristics of Hearing Aids." In 1960 the American National Standards Institute developed a standard S 3.3-1960 entitled "Electroacoustical Characteristics of Hearing Aids." It was revised in 1971, but the revision consisted of a reaffirmation of the 1960 standard. Both documents discuss procedure for measuring the gain, frequency response, and harmonic distortion of hearing aids. They also discuss other elements such as saturation sound pressure level, voltage supply, battery current, etc. The ANSI document and the IEC document are virtually the same in their description of the method of measurement for gain, frequency response curves, and maximum power outputs. They disagree dramatically in their suggested procedures for the measurement of harmonic distortion. IEC suggests an input of 60 dB and an output of 80 dB, while ANSI recommends a 75-dB input and an 80-dB output.

HAIC AND ANSI STANDARDS

The Hearing Aid Industry Conference (HAIC) also made a statement about measurement of hearing aids in 1961. In essence it described a procedure for specifying numerically the frequency response of a hearing aid. This procedure was later also incorporated into an ANSI standards document S 3.8 entitled "Method of Expressing Hearing Aid Performance" in 1967. None of these documents lists any range of acceptability or unacceptability in terms of tolerance or closeness to a standard. Although the HAIC document supports the ANSI procedures document and specifically states that its members will conform to the ANSI procedure, it is interesting to note that this does not appear to be universally true. Both the ANSI and IEC documents, for example, specify that frequency response curves will be measured with a 60-dB input and 100-dB output at 1,000 Hertz. Unfortunately, in most cases, the hearing aid response curves which are provided by the manufacturer were obtained with a 60- to 75-dB input and maximum power output. The latter measurement could give an erroneous impression of the frequency response curve, especially if there were any distortion, which could artifically create an apparent flattening of the frequency response and eliminate hills and valleys. Unfortunately, none of the standards specify such details as the paper speed or pen speed of the graphic level recorder. Yet it is possible to change the written frequency response curve significantly by modifying the pen and paper speed of a graphic level recorder. One study by Kasten and Lotterman (1969) at the Veterans Administration indicated that very few, if any, of the hearing aids which they measured during the course of an investigation yielded frequency response curves which were comparable to those reported as typical by the manufacturer. Part of the problem appeared to be the lack of standard for the exact procedure for running the curve and the fact that the manufacturer may have used a full-on curve rather than the 60 dB in−100 dB out specified by ANSI. It is possible that, since there is no accepted tolerance range standard, the slippage was not considered by the manufacturer.

Use of the Two-Cubic Centimeter Coupler

Another problem which has been under dispute almost since the inception of standards is whether the 2-cc coupler should be used for the measurement of hearing aid performance. Several studies have shown that hearing aids measured with a probe microphone in the human ear yield different values than if that same hearing aid is coupled to a 2-cc coupler. An attempt to solve the problem led to the development of the Zwislocki coupler which appears to more closely approximate the impedance values of the human ear. One manufacturer has developed an artificial head called KEMAR which contains a Zwislocki coupler, thus allowing one to make measurements in an anechoic chamber which reportedly represent the characteristics of that hearing aid on the real ear much more closely than any of the current measurement procedures. However, to develop a standard which would use KEMAR or his equivalent could create undue hardship on some smaller manufacturers.

FDA Standards

These problems have led the Food and Drug Administration to begin to develop the concept of measurement of hearing aids and specifying tolerances. It should be clearly understood that, until the time that the FDA entered into the field of hearing aid measurement, all standards were voluntary. No manufacturer was required by law to measure his hearing aids in the manner suggested by IEC or ANSI or even by the Hearing Aid Industry Conference. The adherence level which was obtained was entirely on a voluntary level.

NEED FOR NEW STANDARDS

The standards which have been developed in the past have only been concerned with a few basic parameters and the procedures for their measurement. However, the characteristics of the measurement apparatus (with the exception of the test environment) have not been specified in great detail, nor have any tolerances been specified. Finally, certain questions were not resolved in the past, such as the difference between the IEC and ANSI standards on the frequencies to be measured for harmonic distortion and the manner in which those frequencies were to be measured.

LITERATURE CITED

Kasten, R., and S. Lotterman, 1969. Influence of hearing aid gain control rotation on acoustic gain. J. Audit. Res. 9: 35–39.

REVIEW OF THE PAST YEAR'S ACTIVITIES IN THE AREA OF HEARING AID STANDARDS

John C. Sinclair

VOLUNTARY STANDARDS

As of May 1975, three voluntary standards were in general use by the hearing aid industry. The most used is ANSI S3.3-1971 (revised from 1960) "Methods for Measurement of Electro-acoustical Characteristics of Hearing Aids." It gives no tolerances nor minimum performance requirements. It does specify the type of coupler and test equipment to be used, i.e., the "standard" 2-cc coupler (HA-2, etc.). It includes recommendations for harmonic distortion measurement and suggests that characteristics such as automatic gain control, noise, intermodulation distortion, telephone-pick-up, and bone conduction have not received general agreement for measurement procedures. This standard parallels closely the International Electrotechnical Commission Publication 118 (1959) "Recommended Methods for Measurements of the Electro-acoustical Characteristics of Hearing Aids," which specifies the measurement of gain, frequency response, tone control, harmonic distortion (at different frequencies than in the ANSI standard), and a measurement of battery current. Finally, there is a short standard S3.8-1967 called "Methods for Expressing Hearing Aid Performance," which specifies an averaging method for arriving at a single number for the gain and output of the hearing aid, generally referred to as the HAIC gain and HAIC output for a hearing aid. This standard also includes a definition of frequency range.

PROBLEMS LEADING TO DEVELOPMENT OF STANDARDS

In December 1973, the Department of Health, Education, and Welfare wrote a letter to the American National Standards Institute asking them to initiate the development of performance and test standards for hearing aids. The Department of Health, Education, and Welfare claimed major problems in the areas of: (1) hearing aids often not meeting quality and performance qualifications; (2) consumers often being given inappropriate and false information on what the hearing aid, as a medical device can do; and (3) keeping instruments used in performing hearing aid evaluations in proper calibration.

The chairman of ANSI S.3 Committee on Bioacoustics wrote back pointing out the complexity of this task because hearing aids were used for a wide variety of impairments and also stated that the characteristics of hearing aids were continually expanded to provide a wide variety of applications. From that time on, statements were issued from the Food and Drug Administration (FDA), to the effect that if medical device performance standards did not originate with nongovernment groups, the federal government would itself have to develop them.

ROLE OF THE FDA IN STANDARDS DEVELOPMENT

In April 1974, another letter came from the Food and Drug Administration of the Department of Health, Education, and Welfare wherein they stated that they "firmly believed that the Hearing Aid Industry Conference working through the American National Standards Committee S-3 could be a viable factor in the development of hearing aid standards," and they asked for a definition of objectives to be carried out over the following year or 18 months and suggested that the following areas be covered: response curves, standards for minimum gain, standards for maximum power output, signal-to-noise ratio, and signal-to-hum ratio. They stated that the standards should not be a deterrent to devices which fall into the "special use" area. The measurements asked for seemed to relate to the National Bureau of Standards measurements made for the Veterans Administration. Therefore, the initial plan during March and April was for the Hearing Aid Industry Conference to work through the

ANSI S3. to develop standards. It is interesting that, at that time, there were 8,000 items to be examined by the FDA on a priority basis and that the hearing aids would eventually work their way up to the top of the list.

HEARING AID INDUSTRY'S RESPONSE TO FDA

It was in March that the Hearing Aid Industry Conference decided definitely that the industry would develop a new standard before FDA action on this matter. They agreed that there was no question that a hearing aid was a medical device and they asked for more input from the FDA; this arrived in July of 1974. The new requirements requested by the FDA were to be in the area of gain, maximum power output, noise, hum, harmonic distortion, intermodulation distortion, compression characteristics, performance versus battery voltage variation, conformation, materials, plug dimensions, marking of control settings, temperature, humidity, shock, and vibration. The hearing aid industry came back with proposals from their Standards Committee, which met for a "final" review in September 1974 in Chicago. During the same period, the FDA had hired an engineer, whose first responsibility was to write a standard for hearing aids for the FDA. The first draft was issued in August 1974. It was quite detailed and, in many areas, followed the untested Canadian standard which had previously been issued in September 1973. The Canadian standard had been criticized by the industry as being partly unworkable, and the FDA draft received the same types of criticisms.

HAIC DISCUSSION PAPER

In September 1974, the HAIC Standards Committee (which includes 15 representatives from the major manufacturers of hearing aids and components) met to review the FDA first draft and to finalize the work that they had been doing on what they called a "discussion paper."

As Chairman of the Standards Committee, I met in September with the FDA to review the first draft and present the HAIC discussion paper. In October 1974, the industrial audiologists were asked to review and comment on the HAIC discussion paper. Also, a well-attended public meeting was held in October. Following the consolidation of these public inputs into the HAIC paper, a meeting was again held with the FDA to review the industry standards. The submission of the industry draft for standards was submitted to the HAIC Board of Directors in December 1974. The Hearing Aid Industry Conference's recommended standards were accepted and approved by the Board in January 1975. These recommendations had some interesting features. For example, they tried to define a minimum gain as the FDA had requested. Although this seems to be a simple point, the minimum performance requirements on output, for example, did not go well with anyone. It is interesting that the FDA were themselves, later in the year, to drop this requirement.

The industry was first to recognize that hearing aids with outputs of greater than 130 dB should be fit with special care simply because one is dealing with maximum saturation sound pressure levels at higher than normal levels. The measurements required were for full-on gain, saturation sound pressure level with 90-dB input, a frequency response curve, tone control effect, saturation control effect, the effect of battery voltage, induction coil sensitivity, the current drain, automatic gain control attack and recovery times, and a small section on harmonic distortion. Many of these had a recommended tolerance associated with them for the first time in any standard on hearing aids. There was a small section on environmental requirements in the areas of temperature, humidity, and vibration, and what turned out to be a fairly complex system for frequency response limits.

FDA Response to HAIC

There was much bickering back and forth during this time. For example, there was a quote in one of the journals, "Implementation of the FDA version of hearing aid standards would impede technical progress, add to consumer cost and create a needless, frustrating, stifling and demoralizing bureaucracy." Nevertheless, the FDA plowed on through drafts two, three, and four, and finally, five was already around in January 1975. The fifth draft was accompanied by a letter asking for comments by March 1975, before publication in the "Federal Register," although legislation was only being considered by Congress to give the FDA regulatory control of medical devices, and, indeed technically, they had no funding provided for the development of standards. The FDA was proceeding on medical device classification by setting up a procedure and establishing classification panels. There are 14 FDA device panels. Hearing aids are covered by the Ear, Nose, and Throat Panel. This panel acts as a classification, proprietary setting, and advisory panel for the FDA.

Classifications of Ear, Nose, and Throat Panel of the FDA

The intent was for the panel to review devices and to permit opportunities for interested persons to submit their views on the classification of a device. The device would be put into one of three classes and, once in that class, would be assigned a priority. The goal was to assure effectiveness and to avoid unreasonable risk of injury or illness. The first classification was life-sustaining or life-supporting devices. The second classification was for devices for which it is appropriate to establish performance standards relating to safety and effectiveness. The third classification was for those devices which were safe and effective when used in conjunction with usage instructions. The hearing aid industry felt that hearing aids should fall into the third classification. Nevertheless, after much debate on this subject, the recommendation of the reviewing panel was that the hearing aids should fall into the second classification.

Industry Response to FDA Panel

It is interesting that the FDA would suggest that they would go into the "Federal Register" without the bill being passed. This threat to publish in the "Federal Register" was a strong one to use on so small an industry as the hearing aid industry. The cost and complexity of compliance to these FDA regulations, once the FDA had published them, hung over our heads. After an initial brush with the FDA, who after all were getting involved in an area admittedly unfamiliar to them, the industry was now on reasonable terms with them. Both were trying to take a realistic approach, although each assumed the other was still unreasonable at this time in certain areas.

Quality Control of Aids

HAIC was invited to the ENT Panel to offer a list of characteristics on hearing aids. I surprised myself when I wrote a "Suggested List of Useful Hearing Aid Characteristics" that it turned out to have 41 characteristics. It was an interesting experience. A question that came at us strongly from the panel was the question of quality control. The panel did not understand quality-price trade-offs. Certainly the industry as a group could not combine on prices in any way or discuss anything that would affect price in any way, such as a "standard" quality. They, like the FDA, did not seem to understand that the cost of perfection can be very high and they were not able to define perfection.

Environmental Tests of Aids

It was, for example, not clear that the added cost of designing a hearing aid to work at $-40°F$ and $+140°F$, as suggested by the FDA drafts, was going to benefit the consumer. Again, would the requirement by the FDA drafts that all technical data accompany the hearing aid (including a schematic) benefit the customer?

REDRAFTING STANDARDS BY THE ANSI COMMITTEE

It was finally decided to get back to the original approach to the problem and that was to have the American National Standards Institute monitor the development of a standard. So the hearing Aid Industry Conference submitted its draft to ANSI S3.48 committee and the FDA submitted their draft to this committee, and S3.48 undertook the task. This committee was under the direction of Sam Lybarger and was a very good committee, well represented by audiology, government, dealers, and manufacturers. The proposed draft was written in May 1975 and was going around for approval vote. We suspected that this draft, in a slightly modified form, would be passed. As a voluntary standard, it could then be used by the FDA, but with additions for environmental testing and format presentation of data, etc.

Presumably, if a medical device bill were passed, the FDA version would be published in the "Federal Register" and legally there would be a 60-day period for anyone to comment.

ANSI's New Method for Measuring Average Gain

Returning to the latest proposed ANSI standard, we note that it covers saturation sound pressure level (SSPL), and includes the warning that if the SSPL is over 132 dB, it must be so noted in the labeling. There is a full-on gain curve interestingly using three different frequencies to get the average gain. These frequencies are 1,000, 1,600, and 2,500. This is an attempt to meet the FDA requirement to parallel as closely as possible the National Bureau of Standards techniques for measuring hearing aids. The NBS uses a "noise" in setting the volume control of a hearing aid for certain measurements. A study was made by the industry which showed that to duplicate this noise system in the various manufacturing plants would be extremely difficult; slight changes in the speakers, the boxes, the absorption, and reflection materials would cause differences in the results obtained. This is carefully documented, and the FDA agreed to this and asked if industry could then find a way of coming up with an equivalent pure tone approach. The choice of these three frequencies gives gains and output very close to those obtained by the National Bureau of Standards' noise measurements. Also, these frequencies are three of the standard recommended frequencies. We have designated this gain as "high frequency gain" to differentiate it from the HAIC gain.

ANSI Method for Setting Reference Gain

In the ANSI recommendations there is a procedure for setting a reference gain, which is reduced volume control setting to allow frequency response, total harmonic distortion, etc. to be measured. There is a new definition of frequency range which is similar, in a sense, to the HAIC frequency range. Total harmonic distortion will be measured with 70-dB input at 500, 800, and 1,600 Hz. This specification will probably have a manufacturer specified maximum tolerance, whereas the gain and saturation sound pressure level will have a plus/minus absolute tolerance associated with it. The equivalent noise, rather than signal-to-noise will be used, and specifics about battery current, induction coil, and AGC measurements will be included.

Estimation of Equipment Tolerances

One of the interesting problems industry has come up with is the tolerances on the equipment used to measure hearing aid parameters. In some cases, these tolerances on the equipment can approach the tolerances desired in the hearing aid characteristics. For example, if the saturation sound pressure level has a ±3-dB absolute tolerance requirement on it and the equipment that we use to measure this in the factory has a ±1-dB tolerance, then manufacturers would actually have to build their hearing aids to within ±2 dB as measured in their factory in order to insure meeting the absolute ±3 dB as required by the standard. This sort of problem occurs continually and is typical of problems which will have to be worked out.

INDUSTRY AND FDA COOPERATION

Finally, a workable consensus type standard may emerge from the American National Standards Institute. The industry is willing to work with the FDA to help assure the public that the consumer receives the best possible product and the most effective and safe product.

PROPOSED AMERICAN NATIONAL STANDARDS INSTITUTE STANDARD FOR SPECIFICATION OF HEARING AID CHARACTERISTICS

Wayne O. Olsen

A new standard defining methods for measuring the electroacoustical characteristics of hearing aids has been proposed by a committee of the American National Standards Institute. The term "proposed standard" occurs here and will be repeated throughout this presentation because the new standard has not been adopted by the American National Standards Institute, as of this time, May, 1975. It has been submitted to another committee, S.3, within the American National Standards Institute for vote. Members of that committee will cast their ballots for or against this document; if all favor it, it will be adopted. If not, the negative votes are to be resolved to the satisfaction of the individuals casting the negative votes, or, failing that, the new standard can be adopted if 80% of the committee favor it. However, an attempt to resolve the difficulties leading to the negative votes must be made before adoption on the basis of an 80% majority. The intent is to obtain unanimous approval if possible.

PURPOSE

Given this background, it is the plan of this paper to present a brief resumé of the proposed standard. In the interest of brevity, the American National

65

Standards Institute is frequently referred to by its acronym, ANSI, in the remainder of this presentation.

PROPOSED STANDARD DEFINES TOLERANCES

The Forward of the proposed standard states that: "This standard is intended to meet the need for specifications of hearing aid performance parameters and their tolerances. The quantities suggested for specification and tolerance are considered to be useful for specifying, selecting or fitting a hearing aid. Use of the methods of specification included in this standard is completely voluntary and discretionary on the part of hearing aid manufacturers or suppliers." The wording here is not unusual except for the mention of tolerances. Previous ANSI documents dealing with hearing aids have delineated methods of measurement, but have not made any recommendations concerning limits or consistency among individual units of a given make and model of hearing aid. Taking cognizance of this new aspect of this proposal, the Forward later states that: "This is the first effort to develop an ANSI hearing aid standard that is directed in part to voluntary tolerances. For this reason, it is recommended that its provisions be widely distributed and evaluated by those affected and that prompt revision be made when deemed needed."

Scope of Proposed Standard

The scope of the proposed standard is set forth in the following statements that: "This standard describes certain hearing aid measurements and parameters that are deemed useful in determining the electro-acoustical performance of a hearing aid. Some of these lend themselves to setting of tolerances for the purpose of maintaining product uniformity and for compliance with the performance specified for a model.

It is not the intention of this document to restrict the variety of hearing aid performance available nor to inhibit in any way advances in the state of the art."

From these statements, it is clear that the proposed ANSI document is not setting minimum requirements for hearing aids; rather, as mentioned earlier, the tolerances given in the document itself are directed at maintaining uniformity among units of given make and model.

High Frequency Average Gain

One major difference in the proposed standard is in the frequencies used for averaging gain and output of the hearing aid. In place of averaging of the usual speech frequencies 500, 1,000, and 2,000 Hz to report hearing aid gain and saturation output, the proposed standard utilizes higher frequencies for averaging, namely, 1,000, 1,600, and 2,500 Hz (Tables 1 and 2). This average, appropriately enough, is labeled the "high frequency" or "HF average" to distinguish it from the 500-, 1,000-, 2,000-Hz average.

Table 1. Measurements

A. High frequency average		
Frequencies	Input	Measurements
1,000, 1,600, and 2,500 Hz	60- or 50-dB SPL	Full-on gain
	90-dB SPL	Saturation sound pressure level (HF average SSPL 90)

B. Reference test gain control position		
Frequencies	Input	Output
1,000, 1,600, and 2,500 Hz	60-dB SPL	Average 17-dB less than HF average SSPL 90 value
(If available gain less than this, full-on gain setting is used.)		

C. Harmonic distortion		
Frequencies	Input	Setting
500, 800, and 1,600 HZ	70-dB SPL	Reference test gain control position

(Omit measurement if frequency response curve shows difference between test frequency and second harmonic > 12 dB.)

D. Equivalent input noise level			
Frequencies	Input	Setting	Measurement
1,000, 1,600, 2,500 Hz	60-dB SPL	Reference test gain control position	HF average output
None		Same	Noise output

Subtract (average output−60) from noise output

continued

Table 1. *continued.*

E. Induction coil sensitivity		
Frequency	Input	Gain control
1,000 Hz	10 mA/m	Full-on
(Hearing aid oriented for highest output.)		

F. AGC characteristics (Input/output function)		
Frequency	Input	Measurement
2,000 Hz	50–90 dB (10-dB steps)	Plot input output curve

(Dynamic characteristics)		
Frequency	Input	Measurement
2,000 Hz	Alternated abruptly between 55 and 80-dB SPL	Attack and release times

G. Specific tolerances	
Measurement	Tolerance
HF average SSPL 90	± 4 dB
HF average full-on gain	± 5 dB
Induction coil sensitivity	± 6 dB
AGC input-output	± 4 dB

H. Manufacturer stated limits	
Measurement	Tolerance
Maximum SSPL 90	Shall not exceed stated value
Harmonic distortion	Shall not exceed stated value
Equivalent input noise level	Shall not exceed stated value
Attack and release times	Within range stated

Use of these frequencies to derive values for gain and saturation output is the result of some work done by the National Bureau of Standards for the Veterans Administration. In testing hearing aids for contract consideration by the V. A., the National Bureau of Standards uses a random noise signal having a long-time average resembling speech to determine saturation

Table 2. Condensed outline of tests being considered in proposed ANSI standard for hearing aid specification[a]

Characteristic	Input SPL dB re 20 μPa	Frequency Hz	Gain control setting	Presentation	Tolerance requirements
SSPL90 (Saturation)	90	200–5,000	Full-on	Curve	Basic test equipment tolerance
Maximum SSPL 90	90	Any frequency between 200 and 5,000	Full-on	Number (dB)	Manufacturer to state maximum value for model
Average SSPL 90	90	1,000, 1,600, 2,500	Full-on	Number (dB) (3-frequency average)	± 4 dB
Average full-on gain	60 or 50 (state which); 50 for AGC	1,000, 1,600, 2,500	Full-on	Number (dB) (3-frequency average)	± 5 dB
Reference test gain control position[b]	60	1,000, 1,600, 2,500	Set gain control back to give output SPL 17 dB less than average SSPL 90, or full-on for low gain aids		17 ± 1 dB
Frequency response	60	200–5,000 or to −20 dB below 3-frequency average	Reference test position	Curve	Low band ± 4 dB; high band ± 6 dB
Total harmonic distortion	70	500, 800, 1,600	Reference test position	Number (%)	Manufacturer to state maximum values for model

continued

Table 2. continued.

Characteristic	Input SPL dB re 20 μPa	Frequency Hz	Gain control setting	Presentation	Tolerance requirements
Equivalent input noise level (L_n)	60	1,000, 1,600, 2,500 (average to get L_{av})	Reference test position	Number (dB) ($L_n - L_2(L_{av} - 60)$)	Manufacturer to state maximum value for model
Telephone pickup induction coil)	10 mA/m rms magnetic field	1,000	Full-on	Number (dB)	Within ± 6 dB of manufacturer's specified value
Battery current	70	1,000	Reference test	Number (mA)	Not to exceed manufacturer's specified maximum for the model
Input-output curves (AGC only)	50–90	2,000	Full-on	Curve input = abcissa; output = ordinate	Match at 70-dB input then to be within ±4 dB of specified
Attack and re-lease times (AGC only)	Abrupt— 55–80; 80–55	2,000	Full-on	Numbers (ms)	To be within values specified by manufacturers

aPrepared by S. F. Lybarger (10-2-75).
bReference test gain control position for AGC aids is full on.

output and in setting gain for other measurements. A series of measurements with the same hearing aids in different facilities quickly revealed that the measurements utilizing such noise signals were not repeatable from facility to facility. This problem appears to be caused by subtle and very difficult to control differences in the noise spectra developed by the test apparatus at the various facilities. It was found, however, that the average of 1,000, 1,600, and 2,500 Hz agreed very well with noise measurements completed at the National Bureau of Standards. Furthermore, the measurements utilizing these tones were repeatable from facility to facility. Consequently, averaging of 1,000, 1,600, and 2,500 Hz was incorporated into the proposed standard rather than the noise measurements originated by the National Bureau of Standards. The 1,000-, 1,600-, and 2,500-Hz frequencies are used to determine the high frequency average full-on gain of an instrument, as measured with gain control full-on and a 60-dB sound pressure level input. (If the hearing aid reaches saturation at the full-on setting and a 60-dB sound pressure level input, a 50-dB sound pressure level input is used instead.)

Measurement of Saturation Sound Pressure Level

These frequencies are also employed to determine the high frequency average saturation sound pressure level. Once again, the gain control of the hearing aid is turned to the full-on setting, but the input signals are at 90-dB sound pressure level. The resultant value is labeled "HF average SSPL 90" for high frequency average saturation sound pressure level, 90-dB input. Additional measurements across the frequency range from 200–5,000 Hz are also completed utilizing the full-on gain setting and a 90-dB sound pressure level input in order to develop a saturation sound pressure level curve. The *top curve* in Figure 1 represents such an SSPL 90 curve.

Reference Test Gain Control Position

Another concept incorporated into the proposed standard that is based on work at the National Bureau of Standards is the "reference test gain control position." This setting is the gain control setting which, with a 60-dB sound pressure level input results in an average output at 1,000, 1,600, and 2,500 Hz that is 17 dB less than that observed with a 90-dB sound pressure level input and full-on gain setting (i.e., the HF average SSPL 90 value). However, if the gain available does not reach a level of 17 dB below the HF average SSPL 90 value, the full-on gain control position is considered the reference test gain control position.

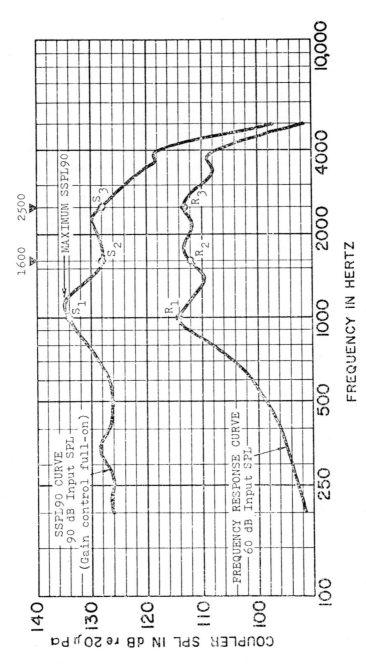

Figure 1. Example of SSPL 90 and frequency response curves. HF-average SSPL 90 = $(S_1 + S_2 + S_3)/3$. Reference test gain control position is determined by: $(S_2 + S_3)/3 - (R_1 + R_2 + R_3)/3 = 17\text{dB}$.

The intent is that the gain control setting for certain tests should be related to the saturation output capability of the hearing aid. "Among the advantages of the gain control setting specified herein are: (1) the gain control is set closer to a typical 'use' setting . . . , (2) harmonic distortion measurements are made with a setting appropriately related to the maximum output capability of the hearing aid, and (3) a reference test gain is specified that is more representative of the 'use' setting than is the 'full-on' gain setting. . . ."

The setting is maintained for frequency response measurements, harmonic distortion measurements, and measurements of equivalent input noise level.

The frequency response curve is measured across the frequency range 200–5,000 Hz with an input level of 60 dB. The lower curve in Figure 1 represents such a frequency response curve.

Harmonic Distortion

Harmonic distortion is measured at 500, 800, and 1,600 Hz with an input level of 70-dB sound pressure level. However, if the frequency response curve reveals a rise of 12 dB or more between a distortion test frequency and its second harmonic, distortion tests at that frequency may be omitted.

Internal Noise

The equivalent input noise level measurement in essence is a determination of the internal noise of the hearing aid. For it, the hearing aid output without any signal input is measured; the reference test gain (determined earlier as 17 dB below the HF average SSPL 90 value, or, as mentioned earlier, full-on gain for some instruments) is then subtracted from the internal noise measurement of the hearing aid and recorded as the equivalent input noise level.

Induction Coil

Among additional measurement procedures described in the proposed standard is the measurement of the sensitivity of the induction coil, i.e., the telephone pickup of the hearing aid. The hearing aid is placed in the magnetic field developed by a 1,000-Hz 10 mA/m rms current and its output is measured with the gain control set to the full-on position.

Automatic Gain Control

Measurements of automatic gain control (AGC) hearing aids are also described in the proposed standard. Saturation output and full-on gain are measured in the same manner as hearing aids not having automatic gain control circuitry. In addition, hearing aid output is plotted as function of increasing a 2,000-Hz input signal from 50- to 90-dB sound pressure level in steps small enough to determine the action of the AGC circuit. A 2,000-Hz tone is also utilized to evaluate the dynamic characteristics of the AGC circuitry. With the hearing aid gain control in the full-on position, the 2,000-Hz input is alternated abruptly between the levels of 55-dB sound pressure level and 80-dB sound pressure level. The output of the hearing aid is observed on an oscilloscope to measure the attack and release times of the AGC circuit. "The attack time is defined as the time between the abrupt increase from 55 to 80 dB and the point where the level is within 2 dB of the steady state value for the 80-dB input. The release time is defined as the interval between the abrupt drop from 80 to 55 dB and the point where the signal is within 2 dB of the steady state value for the 55-dB input sound pressure level."

Tolerances

Turning now to the tolerances mentioned earlier, the proposed standard suggests specific tolerances for saturation, full-on gain, the frequency response curve, the sensitivity of the telephone pickup coil, and AGC characteristics.

Saturation Output

Related to the saturation output of the hearing aid, it is suggested that the HF average SSPL 90 (high frequency average of 1,000, 1,600, and 2,500 Hz with 90-dB sound pressure level input) be within ±4 dB of the value specified by the manufacturer for that model. In other words, it is suggested that each unit of that particular model develop an HF average SSPL 90 within 4 dB of that reported by the manufacturer.

Insofar as full-on gain is concerned, the proposed standard suggests that the high frequency average full-on gain of each hearing aid of a given model be within ± 5 dB of the value specified by the manufacturer for that model.

Similarly, it is suggested that the output of the hearing aid switched to the telephone coil pickup be within ±6 dB of the value specified by the manufacturer.

The proposed standard suggests that tolerances for the frequency response curve be determined in the following manner. Figure 2 shows the following steps for determining the band width and tolerances:

1. From the manufacturer's specified frequency response curve, determine the average of the 1,000-, 1,600-, and 2,500-Hz coupler sound pressure level values.
2. Subtract 20 dB.
3. Draw a horizontal line at the reduced level.
4. Note the lowest frequency, f_1, at which the response curve intersects the straight line.
5. Note the highest frequency, f_2, at which the response curve intersects the straight line if this is less than 5,000 Hz.
6. The tolerance range is then defined as being from 1.25 f_1 to 4,000 Hz, or 0.8 f_2 if less than 4,000 Hz.

Two tolerance bands are indicated: the low band with frequency limits of 1.25 f_1 to 2,000 Hz has a tolerance of ±4 dB; and the high band with frequency limits of 2,000 to 0.8 f_2 Hz but not more than 4,000 Hz has a tolerance of ±6 dB. Compliance with the tolerances suggested above may be made using a suitable template with upper and lower limit curves that are derived from the manufacturer's specified response curve for the model.

Vertical adjustment of the template on the response curve of the measured hearing aid is permitted.

Horizontal adjustment up to 10% in frequency is permitted.

Suggested tolerances for other hearing aid characteristics are specified by the manufacturer. The statement "should not exceed that specified for the model" (i.e., specified by the manufacturer) is used to define the tolerance for harmonic distortion and equivalent input noise level.

Tolerances for the AGC characteristics of a given model state that its output for 50 and 90 dB SPL input should not deviate from that specified by the manufacturer by more than ±4 dB. With regard to the attack and release times, they should be with ±5 msec or ±50%, whichever is greater, of the values specified by the manufacturer for that model.

There are, of course, numerous other facets in the proposed standard dealing with the test apparatus, the test space, and calibration, but it was the purpose of this presentation to concern itself only with the electroacoustic measurements of hearing aids as described in the document under consideration.

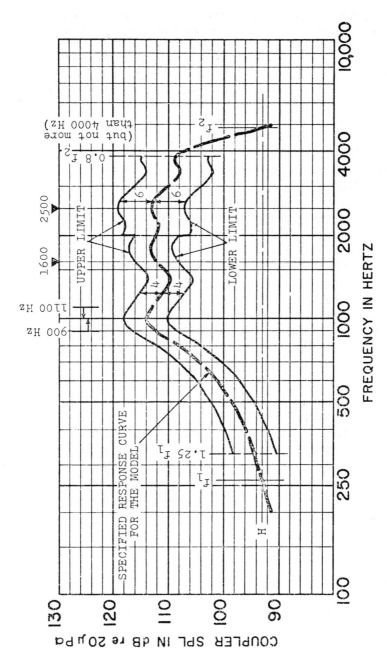

Figure 2. Example of construction of tolerance template for frequency response curve. Horizontal line H is 20 dB below the average of the 1,000, 1,600, and 2,500 Hz levels on the specified response curve. In use, the template must be kept square with the graph on the measured curve, but may be adjusted vertically any amount and horizontally up to ±10% in frequency. Lines on the template at 900 and 1,100 Hz show the maximum allowable horizontal movement referred to the 1,000-Hz ordinate on the measured curve. After adjustment of the template, the measured curve must lie between the upper and lower limits on the template.

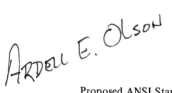

SUMMARY OF PROPOSED STANDARDS

To summarize, a new standard describing procedures for measuring hearing aids has been proposed by the committee of the American National Standards Institute. This proposal was being considered and was voted upon by another committee within ANSI. The proposed standard differs from previous ANSI standards dealing with hearing aids in that different frequencies are used to determine average saturation output, full-on gain, and, in the use of a defined reference test, gain control setting when determining the frequency response, harmonic distortion, and equivalent input noise level of the hearing aid. In addition, the proposed standard also describes measurement procedures for the telephone coil pickup and the automatic gain control characteristics of the instrument. The proposed standard also indicates tolerances for various characteristics in order to define product uniformity for a given make and model of hearing aid.

DISCUSSION

ELECTROACOUSTIC PARAMETERS

AUDIENCE MEMBER: During the discussion of the proposed standard, was polar response or directional response considered?

DR. OLSEN: There has been lots of discussion, but there is nothing in the proposed document about polar response.

AUDIENCE MEMBER: Does the battery current also include the maximum drain of the battery?

BATTERY CHARACTERISTICS

DR. OLSEN: We are not clear on the battery characteristics yet. The battery current will be measured with full-on gain setting, 60-dB input at 1 K. A tolerance will be put on that also. The tolerances that were put on the hearing aid parameters are as seen here. The HF average full-on gain is within ±5 dB and is relative to the value specified by the manufacturer for that unit. All the numbers are relative to those specified by the manufacturer for that given model. Saturation sound pressure level is within ±4 dB. The induction coil sensitivity (the telephone coil pickup) is ±6 dB at 1,000 Hz.

ABSOLUTE TOLERANCES

DR. SINCLAIR: These are absolute tolerances. Specifically, the gauge is ±5 dB from an absolute value. That means that if one is going to (1) build a hearing aid or (2) measure a hearing aid, tolerances have to be subtracted from that number. If I had 2-dB tolerances in the engineering specifications, as a manufacturer, I would have to build the aid to ±3 dB. That's a very critical point. In other words, these proposals are absolute tolerances which include the equipment tolerances. Some people claim they are large, but for manufacturers who are going to have to tighten their equipment standards to build hearing aids, that is a very tight tolerance.

PROBLEMS OF MEASURING TOLERANCES

DR. OLSEN: There is ±1 dB on the mike used to monitor the sound field. There is ±1 dB on the mike that picks up the output from the hearing aid. Thus, you have 2 dB on those two mikes. Therefore, the manufacturer has to hold within ±4 dB to achieve the ±6 dB accepted tolerance.

AUDIENCE MEMBER: Under the best possible conditions at one frequency, it is great to achieve a repeat measurement of ±0.7 dB.

DR. SINCLAIR: Let's just pursue the argument to where it ultimately might go. If a hearing aid is manufactured at facility A and then the FDA gets into the act and says, "Hearing aids have to perform within certain tolerances or they will not be certified," one then really has four mikes with which to contend. There are the two mikes at the manufacturer and the two mikes at the FDA.

AUDIENCE MEMBER: The difficulty is not going to be with the mikes. It's going to be with the test chamber. The mikes are likely to be accurate because they can be calibrated rather precisely and allowances may be easily made for their deviation.

DR. OLSEN: Remember we are not talking about one facility, we are talking about two facilities and two sets of equipment.

If we are now going to measure a hearing aid, what do we do? What are our tolerances? If the tolerance were an absolute number and I gave you the aid and I asked you to measure it, you would have to add your equipment tolerances to the allowable aid tolerance. You don't know that I am building an aid to a ±5 dB tolerance. It could be 5 dB from absolute with the aid I give you. To check that, you are going to have to add to your equipment tolerances to include that 5 dB. Going in that direction you might be measuring ± 7 dB. We discussed this concept for hours. We have put down the absolute values here and we're going to see how the equipment goes. This is an interpretation which nearly killed us. This measurement tolerance has to hold in Denver and in Washington. The aid can be made in Denver and tested in Washington, but it has to hold to certain standards. There is no correction factor for a difference in altitudes, which will play havoc with directional hearing aids.

PROBLEMS IN MEASURING FREQUENCY RESPONSE AND AGC

DR. OLSEN: The frequency response measurement also has tolerances which should be discussed. For the frequency range below 2,000 Hz, the frequency tolerance is 40 Hz, and for the frequency range about 2,000 Hz, the frequency is ±60 Hz. There is also the problem of determining the frequency response (or the band width) of the hearing aid. Under the old documents one measures the average of 500, 1,000, and 2,000 Hz, then drops down and draws a line across the frequency response curve. In the new document one uses the HF average and the reference test gain control position, then drops down 20 dB and draws a line through the point. The point where a horizonal line intercepts is the frequency response or the band width of the hearing aid. Remember, there is a tolerance of 1.25 times the frequency which is acceptable for the low end of the response curve and 0.8 for the high end of the curve. Again, the tolerance refers to the number specified by the manufacturer for that particular hearing aid. This is the tolerance on the frequency response of the hearing aid. The big difference is that it is 20 dB down from the high frequency average and the fact that there is a tolerance specified for it. In addition, the harmonic distortion should not exceed the value specified by the manufacturer. The noise input level should not exceed that specified by the manufacturer as well.

The AGC characteristics which the manufacturer sets for bands or boundaries on the hearing aid should fall within those boundaries. When the frequency response 90-dB curve exceeds 130-dB output, the hearing aid has to be marked. The instructional manual, the data sheet, and the hearing aid itself have to indicate that the aid is intended for severe hearing loss cases. There is also a caution statement, that, if 130 dB is exceeded, the following statement must be enclosed: "Special care must be exercised in the treating of hearing aids with maximum sound pressure levels greater than 130 dB, as there may be damage to residual hearing of the hearing impaired." That is approximately the statement that is to be put into the proposed document.

Notice that part of the discussion regarding setting tolerances here for frequency response, distortion, and power output is relative to the manufacturer's specifications. This allows a competitive edge. If the standards use a small number on distortion, then the manufacturers are going to compete to provide aids with that small number. If a big number on the gain is wanted, then the manufacturers could compete for that big number. In this particular document, leaving what the hearing aid does up to the manufacturer and then only asking him to provide aids whose numbers are within the specified tolerances does keep the competition in there.

STANDARDS ON CORDS

AUDIENCE MEMBER: Are there standards on cords?

DR. SINCLAIR: On body aids, all cords and plugs must be uniform. That is going to hurt some manufacturers. The small little pins that some manufacturers use would not be acceptable to the FDA. As designers, we don't like it for we don't like to be restricted in design. Audiologists tend to like it because they want to be able to easily replace the cords, but it may be that some future design possibility is being thrown away. If cords are standardized, improvements cannot come. I hope that's not a weak argument, but that's the argument designers have been using.

HEARING AID REPAIRS

AUDIENCE MEMBER: Is this for new aids only or for repaired aids also?

DR. SINCLAIR: I would interpret it that the repaired aid must come back meeting the standard.

DR. OLSEN: Are repairs part of the FDA document?

DR. SINCLAIR: If the FDA asks for all this information to go with the aid, it brings up the question of repair. How do manufacturers control that aid? How then does the person who repairs it bring it back to that specification unless he has a copy of the specification?

DR. OLSEN: That is getting into type approval. John, please explain what is meant by a type approval versus a certification.

FDA TYPE APPROVAL OF HEARING AIDS

DR. SINCLAIR: The FDA has swung back and forth. At the moment, they are talking about using type approval, which means that a manufacturer can get a model approved. The definition of a model is a little tighter. The adjustability of the aid comes into question. If there is a control inside the aid or battery compartment that the user cannot change but the audiologist or dealer can change, then what model is being tested? The FDA is not clear as to how they are going to get around that. Type approval would be the simplest one. Industry could get type approval to produce an aid and all aids with that model name would have to meet the standard. Users would then go to a clinic or a store and purchase the particular aid and test it to the factory model type. It is not yet the law to do this.

DR. OLSEN: The funds have not been appropriated yet.

DR. SINCLAIR: They do have 105 people sitting around to do all of this. They are in existence. If the aid does not meet the stated parameters, the FDA will tell the manufacturer that he must stop producing that aid. Apparently the aids would be recalled if they fail to meet these standards.

DR. WILBER: Isn't that what the FDA does with some kinds of products already?

DR. SINCLAIR: Yes, with drugs.

DR. WILBER: Won't this approach perhaps make the manufacturer a little more careful about what he says that his models will do?

DR. SINCLAIR: Truth in advertising will come out of this.

DR. WILBER: Right now the only thing an audiologist can do if a manufacturer says an aid can do a particular thing and it can't is to try to get him for false advertising.

DR. SINCLAIR: It is true that now the Federal Trade Commission (FTC) will get after him. There is a little bit of an argument now between the FDA and the FTC about jurisdictional responsibility. They are fighting about who is in charge of what which makes me a little pleased.

DR. OLSEN: The point is that the measurements that the FDA makes the manufacturer present describe the internal control settings that are used. Then the FDA makes the measurement according to what the manufacturer has described.

AUDIENCE MEMBER: Can't the manufacturer just change the specifications so that he can meet it?

DR. SINCLAIR: No, no! Once industry gets approval on the specifications for a particular model, they are not allowed to change it.

AUDIENCE MEMBER: Suppose they just say, "This is a new model." Then it goes to the FDA where it is tested. If it turns out that it is out of line, the manufacturer can change the printed specifications.

ARGUMENTS AGAINST FDA REGULATIONS

DR. SINCLAIR: Industry must still deal within *model specifications*. It would have to be a different model. Remember the Nader report? The thing that everyone kept hearing was, "Why are they picking on the hearing aid industry?" The Nader report had a horrible name, "Paying through the ear," a couple of years back.

The FDA doesn't seem to be asking itself loudly enough, "What am I doing for the person who must wear the aid? Why do I measure at 122° and 95% relative humidity?" If it is going to cost a good deal to buy the equipment to make those measurements (which it will), it is naive to think that the manufacturer, or even the distributor, is going to absorb the costs. The FDA never asks the question, "What is it going to cost the final purchaser of the hearing aid?" Aids are expensive now; think what this might do.

DR. WILBER: Maybe that argument should be made more strongly to the FDA.

DR. SINCLAIR: It's been heard. For the uniformity in product and for the advertisement, I think it is good. The FDA asked industry what it was going to cost. On the spur of the moment, I told them!

We were at an eyeglass meeting in Washington with the VA. The opening statement that Don Causey made was that the VA buys from 45 manufacturers. A lot of those must be small manufacturers. The big companies can survive. The question is, "What about the small companies?" It's antitrust and anticompetitive.

DR. OLSEN: To assure that hearing aids meet the requirements, a lower number like 128 dB will have to be accepted and then all aids above that will be marked. That's going to happen.

MEDICAL CLEARANCE

DR. SINCLAIR: In April 1975, the industry adopted as a policy the concept of medical clearance. In other words, the industry is saying one should get a clearance from a doctor before being fitted with a hearing aid.

If we had gotten in the third classification everything would have been voluntary. We wouldn't be talking about mandatory standards. We are in classification two. We are medical devices. The audiologists are heavily involved in the discussion of medical prescriptive devices in many states.

DR. WILBER: Audiologists are thinking that there must be two kinds of clearances—medical and audiological.

EXPECTED LIFE OF A HEARING AID

AUDIENCE MEMBER: Please comment on the life of a hearing aid.

DR. SINCLAIR: An average life for a hearing aid statistically, of all the 600,000 hearing aids sold in the United States, is 3.3 years. The FDA is requiring in this standard that parts of a hearing aid be maintained for 6 years. They have been asking for a 5-year life. The VA is expecting a

5-year life. In reality, the statistics show a 3.3-year life. That's how often people change their aids.

DR. WILBER: That's a totally different thing. There are patients who have been told by their hearing aid dealer that they have had that aid for 2 years and now it's time to get a new one.

DR. SINCLAIR: As a personal observation, if I owned an aid I would trade it after 5 years. It's very much like most consumer products. After 5 years, things just start to go, like rubber parts, and manufacturers know of no way of stopping it. There are many, many more aids going past that 3.3-year average. People are asking that industry clean their aid, fix it, and keep it going. In our company we are seeing people holding on to their aids much longer now. Our company is getting a lot more requests for reconditioning. However, aids may be difficult to repair after 5 years.

AUDIENCE MEMBER: Have you any idea what the failure rate is on the hearing aid?

DR. SINCLAIR: The mean time between failures for each component has been asked by the hearing aid industry. "How long can we keep an aid going? What can be said for each component in the aid? That is: What is the mean time between failures?" The component suppliers just will *not* go along on that at this time. Manufacturers can't get that information from suppliers.

The total annual sales for the industry is 600,000 aids. That is a very small volume for a manufacturer selling resistors or capacitors. The manufacturer who makes millions of resistors and capacitors doesn't want to run the risk of having the government step into his plant and say, "You sold the hearing aid industry these, and the failure rate is too high." They don't want to have the government sticking its nose in their business.

RELATIONSHIP OF MEDICAL
CLEARANCE AND HEARING AID DISPENSING

AUDIENCE MEMBER: A while back, you said the industry is in favor of medical clearance. How do the hearing aid dealers relate to that?

DR. SINCLAIR: In most cases dealers are independent businessmen. They sell hearing aids. They sell anybody's hearing aids. Some of the companies say, "Don't let these people get to a doctor. Tell them they need an aid." That's wrong. Industry would like to create the feeling that if a person needs a hearing aid, he should first see a doctor. Maybe industry should be saying, "Go to see your audiologist—or see both." The medical clearance that industry wants their association members to use is to encourage patients to see a doctor. Maybe audiologists should get back to industry and get them to say, "Go see both a physician and an audiologist." The other day someone came to us and asked to see me. He had fallen off a ladder the week before and lost his hearing. He wanted a hearing aid. I told him to see a doctor.

DR. WILBER: Is the industry specifying any type cf doctor?

DR. SINCLAIR: No, we don't specify.

DR. OLSEN: I thought I saw a draft of the NADS statement that said: "Someone who specializes in ear diseases."

DR. SINCLAIR: Some of the states specify that a dealer must have a signature that the client has seen a doctor before he can sell them a hearing aid, especially for a certain age group.

DR. WILBER: There is a movement now to increase that age factor.

DR. SINCLAIR: Or you can get a waiver.

DR. WILBER: California has a waiver, but they are trying to get rid of it.

DR. OLSEN: Some of the states have a waiver to the effect of: "I have read or have had read to me this particular waiver and I choose not to see a physician." However, there is no provision for signing the waiver outside the age limit between 16 and 60. Beyond these age limits, the doctor's signature is mandatory.

FDA AND HEARING AID MEASUREMENTS

AUDIENCE MEMBER: Do you think the FDA will require hearing aid dealers to do some measurements on the hearing aid, like distortion measurement, gain, etc?

DR. SINCLAIR: The FDA would like to eliminate all measurements made by the dealer. The dealer becomes a salesman or disperser, so the answer would be, "No."

One of the problems that is coming up—but which hasn't hit the industry yet—is that a lot of people are buying these small test boxes. The correlation from box to box is not the same. Some audiologists are buying them and measuring hearing aids and drawing all sorts of conclusions. It has caused a lot of problems.

DR. WILBER: There are some measurements that one can use the small boxes for, however, One must know what it can or cannot do.

AUDIENCE MEMBER: The problem is that the accoustical environment is relatively poor within the box. The instrumentation is accurate, but the particle velocity and wave velocity are different. The accuracy of the field is not very well described. In order to get a decent accoustical environment, the laws of physics cannot be revoked.

SUMMARY

Laura Ann Wilber

PROMULGATION OF STANDARDS

In summary, a great deal of information was presented on the specifics of the proposed FDA regulations and of the proposed new ANSI standard with special emphasis on those areas which will be different from the old ANSI standard. As may be observed, the emphasis seems to be changing from the simple requirement that hearing aids should be measured, to the promulgation of standards which specify the particulars of the way in which hearing aids must be measured. There may be additional regulations requiring the manufacturer to adhere to certain standards. The usefulness of any standard is only as good as the persons using and interpreting it. Therefore, it is important for audiologists not only to be familiar with current hearing aid standards, but also to understand their meaning and the potential import of each standard on the performance of the aid as it applies to the patient with a hearing loss.

AUDIOLOGICAL RESPONSIBILITY TOWARDS STANDARDS

The FDA standard is printed in the "Federal Register" when an agreement is reached, and the ANSI standard is available from the American National Standards Institute, 1430 Broadway, New York, New York. It is also possible that the ANSI standard may be printed by the Acoustical Society of America. Any Hearing Aid Industry Conference standard is available directly from the hearing aid industry and may be printed in a publication such as the "Hearing Aid Journal." It probably behooves all professionals to make certain that they do have the most current standards and that, when measurements of hearing aids are performed in clinics, adherence to the standard procedures is followed just as closely as the manufacturer is expected to do in his plant.

HISTORICAL DEVELOPMENT OF STANDARDS

Dr. Sinclair, representing industry, traced the history of the development of standards for the measurement of hearing aids. He observed then that, in 1959, the IEC, an international group, developed procedures for the measurement of hearing aids. Subsequently, ANSI also developed standards, and finally the industry itself—the Hearing Aid Industry Con-ference—developed some standards for measurement. However, all of these organizations and bodies were voluntary. That meant that anybody, any company wishing to use the standards proposed by these organizations, might do so, but no one was required to do so. In addition, these groups developed standards which only told one *how* to measure, not what interpretation or what leniency or variability should be allowed in the measurement. Dr. Sinclair indicated that everyone is faced with a different type of problem because the FDA may impose standards for tolerance. If a company produced a given model, that model must adhere, within certain ranges, to the standard which has been set for that instrument. This was a new approach and a new angle. It would be a matter of government control which might or might not be good. That issue was discussed and not totally resolved because it really was beyond our jurisdiction. But, it's going to happen!

DEVELOPMENT OF NEW STANDARDS

Dr. Olsen described the ongoing work of a committee of the American National Standards Institute, which was also trying to develop new standards for the measurement of hearing aids. These standards also set limitations. This committee has been very clever and they have invited an FDA man to work with the ANSI group in order to effect some communication between the working groups. ANSI standards groups are open: anyone can go and listen to the committees, and can contribute if the chairman allows them to do so. This particular group was composed of audiologists and members of industry.

PROPOSED STANDARDS

There was broad input into the ANSI standards group. Dr. Olsen spoke about some of the proposed standards. One which would be of interest was the development of a frequency response curve which was a high frequency response curve or a high frequency gain measurement. In the past we have talked about HAIC gains being the average of 500, 1,000, and 2,000 Hz. If this new standard passed, the high frequency gain would be the average of 1,000, 1,600, and 2,500 Hz. Reasoning backward as to why these particular numbers were used, we realized that part of it had to do with the frequency spectrum and the slope of speech. In the past, many high frequency emphasis aids have been given misleading gain figures because HAIC gain estimates were based on averaging 500, 1,000, and 2,000 Hz.

NEED FOR AUDIOLOGICAL INPUT

Dr. Olsen reported that a new ANSI proposed standard covered distortion at 500, 800, and 1,600 Hz and a saturation SPL curve at 90-dB input. All of these were new ideas and there were many more in the proposed current standard. On the other hand, the proposed FDA standards for the measurement of hearing aids and for their tolerances were published in June 1975. I believe it is the responsibility of audiologists to respond. We can write directly to the federal government. We need to tell them what we think is good and what we think is poor in relation to the proposed standard. If we do not, and if there are no reactions, then whatever the government decrees will go into effect. I feel quite certain that people around the country will be responding.

It is comparatively easy to measure hearing aids because one has to use equipment and not people at all. One can manipulate equipment in ways that one can never manipulate people. These were some of the areas discussed in trying to solve the problem of how to measure hearing aids.

HEARING AIDS
FOR
INFANTS
AND
CHILDREN

INTRODUCTION

Martha Rubin

The rationale for making assumptions about hearing-impaired children stems from observations of hearing children. Sometimes the generalization from hearing to hearing impaired, however, is not a good fit. There is a need to observe the hearing-impaired child in his *own* environment in order to examine the intactness of his sensory and linguistic analyzers, to prevent secondary emotional problems, and to allow the child's innate preprograming for language to progress in an optimal atmosphere.

NORMAL INFANT RESEARCH

Interest in the hearing child has been whetted in the last 5 years by exciting research demonstrating that the hearing infant is ready at birth to respond to human language. Recently, Cairns and Butterfield (1974) showed that hearing infants, 12 hours after birth, indicated their preferences for *singing* voices rather than for white noise. On the first day of life, Condon and Sander (1973) filmed the synchronous gestures of hearing infants in a hospital nursery who assumed a typical posture to the word "come" when the nurse said, "Come and see who's over here." Infant research dates back to about 1971 when Eimas demonstrated that 1-month-old infants were responsive to speech sounds /pa/ and /ba/, and were able to discriminate between them in a linguistically relevant manner. Four-month-old infants were shown by Kaplan (1969) to discriminate intonational contours and stress patterns. In other words, hearing infants are developing listening skills from the day they are born. Their innate disposition for language, according to Chomsky (1965), needed only to be triggered by the environment. Eisenberg (1976) presented basic research in this area.

IMPLICATIONS FOR HEARING-IMPAIRED INFANTS

The implications for hearing-impaired infants are quite clear. First, there is a need for identification of hearing loss during the first 3 months of life and, secondly, there is a responsibility to provide *appropriate amplification* within the first *few* months of life. Audiological judgment to recommend amplification is based on a number of variables—type and severity of loss, etiology of loss, parental cooperation, and most importantly, the availability of a total habilitative program. Hearing-impaired infants require ongoing audiological monitoring in an educational millieu.

LITERATURE CITED

Cairns, G. F., and E. C. Butterfield. 1974. Assessing infants' auditory functioning. *In* B. Z. Friedlander (ed.), Exceptional Infant. Vol. II, pp. 84–108.

Chomsky, N. 1965. Aspects of the Theory of Syntax. Massachusetts Institute of Technology Press, Cambridge, Mass. pp. 47–59.

Condon, S. W., and L. W. Sander. 1973. Neonate movement is synchronized with adult speech: Interactional participation and language acquisition. Science 183: 99–101.

Eisenberg, R. B. 1976. Auditory Competence in Early Life. University Park Press, Baltimore.

Kaplan, E. L. 1969. The role of intonation in the acquisition of language. Unpublished doctoral dissertation. Cornell University, Ithaca, N. Y.

HEARING AIDS FOR INFANTS AND TODDLERS

Martha Rubin

Many of the babies evaluated at the Lexington Hearing Center were referred by virtue of their being in a "high risk category" defined by the Joint Committee on Infants Screening in 1975. Ehrlich et al. (1973) showed that birth history may raise suspicions about possible hearing loss. Etiologies such as prematurity, maternal rubella, hereditary hearing loss, congenital abnormality, and neurological impairment may result in hearing loss. According to Curlee's report (1975), approximately 6% of all live births *should be* assigned to a high risk register.

HEARING-IMPAIRED BABIES AT THE LEXINGTON SCHOOL FOR THE DEAF

The babies evaluated at our center demonstrating hearing loss ranged in age from 1 month to 3 years. They were followed co-jointly in our Hearing Center and in our Infant Center.

In 1974 we had six babies under 6 months, four under a year, and 16 toddlers under 3 years of age. Of the 26 children, 10 had deaf parents. That was an understandable statistic since we were part of the Lexington School for the Deaf and deaf parents may have felt more comfortable there than in a hospital setting. Etiology among our six infants was congenital deafness in two cases, meningitis in one case, rubella in one case, and unknown in two cases who were referred by astute pediatricians. Our older babies' etiologies included one Down's syndrome. There were several multiply handicapped toddlers in whom the effects of hearing loss were intensified considerably by mental retardation, emotional disturbance, and neurological impairment.

Team Approach for Infants

Strategies for diagnostic and habilitative measures differed according to the needs and capacities of each mother-child diad, but there was one aspect of our program common to each diad—that is, each was part of a total habilitative matrix in which mother and child interacted with a variety of communicating professionals. The Infant Center *teacher* acted as liason and was physically present during *all* diagnostic and habilitative sessions—while audiologists also observed the baby in the Infant Center nursery weekly.

Castle and Ventry (1967) showed that a team approach was necessary for the 3-year old who was tested and fitted with aids in the speech and hearing hospital center. In New York, the passage of the Baby Bill in February 1973 shifted the responsibility for the deaf infant somewhat from the hospital to the school, and new programs of comprehensive health care were being carefully developed in an *educational* environment throughout the state.

In any setting, health care is critical for the tiny infant who has only recently been physically separated from the mother. The mother's needs are critical as well. When she learns that her baby is defective, she is more vulnerable to depression than the mother of an older child who has had time to develop defenses. The mother-child relationship during the first 6 months may influence the ego development of the child and his relationship to the world later on. The responsibility for this emerging mother-child relationship was united among many disciplines at Lexington—pediatric, otological, nursing, social work, special education, and audiology. In this setting, since all disciplines were physically close, communication was direct and fast. In this setting, the needs of the hearing-impaired infant and toddler were special.

CLINICAL TESTING OF BABIES

In what ways are babies' audiological needs special? First, clinical methods of testing a young baby were limited to behavioral audiometry, visual reinforcement audiometry, and impedance testing. New techniques such as electrocochleography, respiration audiometry, and brainstem audiometry were still in an experimental state. At the Lexington Hearing Center, three audiologists, an Infant Center teacher, and the baby's parents observed the baby's responses in the soundproof booth. Stimuli were warbled pure tones and speech, and retest was scheduled within 1 week. Babies were *always* given priority scheduling, but the retest appointment depended on the child. Usually, retesting 1 hour before feeding was a good rule (Eisenberg, 1970). Impedance testing was scheduled directly before medication time. For example, if a baby was medicated with phenobarbital three times a day, it was tested directly before the afternoon medication because phenobarbital may relax the stapedius muscle reflex. In cases where the amount of medication was unknown, blood samples could be drawn to ascertain the amount of the drug present. Those hearing-impaired babies who were on long-term medication needed to have the maximum power output of the hearing aid reduced because their stapedius muscle reflex was not functioning in a defensive way against noise.

High Incidence of Serous Otitis Media in Infants

Another area in which the hearing-impaired infant was special appeared to be the high incidence of middle ear pathology. Porter (1974) reported an incidence of 23% of middle ear pathology among school age children in the Kansas School for the Deaf. Last year 50% of the children in the Lexington Infant Center had demonstrated middle ear pathology. Our sample consisted of 16 infants and toddlers. Six babies had deaf parents and 10 babies had hearing parents. In each group of deaf and hearing parents, half of the babies had otitis media or serous otitis media at least once. Five babies of hearing parents had recurrent episodes necessitating myringotomies and tubal implantation. Thus, *no* difference was observed between the abilities of deaf and hearing parents to identify middle ear problems, but deaf infants of hearing parents appeared to have more middle ear problems. All of these infants required *ongoing* impedance testing *during* hearing aid fitting to rule out fluctuating hearing loss. An audiologist has to be certain the baby's ears function well when real ear aid measurements are taken as a basis of hearing aid performance with a specific hearing aid.

Physical Problems of Fitting Aids on Infants

The third reason why hearing-impaired infants were special was because they have tiny ears. This factor necessitated several unusual audiological procedures if ear-level aids were to be recommended. One was that the criteria for choice of an aid could depend on the shape of the aid, or the location of the microphone, as well as on the electroacoustical characteristics. Thicker aids tend to distort a baby's helix and antihelix, resulting in a "lop" ear effect. Aids with a top microphone appear to reduce acoustical feedback. Second, earmolds need to be replaced frequently, in order to maintain that elusive goal—a good acoustic seal. Third, tape was needed to keep the ear-level aid securely in place. It is hoped that manufacturers will accept some of the recommendations made by the Academy of Rehabilative Audiology's 1973 Task Force Report on hearing aids for children, so that a more suitable aid for babies can be designed and manufactured.

ELECTROACOUSTIC CHARACTERISTICS OF ACCEPTABLE AIDS

Electroacoustically, babies may have different acoustic needs than do older children. Successful aiding for babies depends on knowledge of *their* acoustic environment and on the available perceptual clues in the acoustic signals they receive.

Lexington's stringent preselection criteria for the aids chosen for infants and toddlers eliminate excessive distortion and low output from the aids in the infant inventory, as well as other inventories. We never relied on manufacturers' specification data. Each aid was analyzed in *our* anechoic chamber. Ear-level aids were chosen with minimal harmonic distortion of under 10%. Acoustic analysis showed that ear-level aids were as powerful as any body-worn instruments and quite suitable for deaf children when not driven to saturation. Martoni and Reisberg of Sweden and Reilly of Australia (Personal communications) wrote that ear-level aids were being used extensively in their countries. Infants at Lexington used ear-level aids since 1973 and were regarded by staff and parents as the single most important habilitative tool available to an educational facility. Recent ear-level aids can provide amplification through 7,000 Hz and can be selectively adjusted.

Hearing Aids for Deaf Parents of Deaf Infants

In 1975 a unique program for unaided deaf parents of Infant Center babies was added. Ten sets of deaf parents who had not used aids in at least 12 to 15 years were evaluated for hearing aids and given hearing aids through a special grant. The next step was auditory training. Only one parent started a formal programed instruction auditory training course, but the other parents learned to listen along with their babies. Among 10 mothers, only one refused to use an aid because of trauma as a young girl. Deaf parents reported that, for the first time, they had heard and responded to their child's cries for help or to their baby's vocalizations (Rubin, Rubin, and Jupiter, 1975).

In a recent study, Greenstein (1975) analyzed the *traits* of *hearing* mothers of deaf children which correlated highly with good language skills of their children at age 3. He found that the two traits with the highest correlations were: (1) the ability to motivate without coercion and (2) the ease in managing her child. Deaf mothers would be better able to manage their children if they could *hear* their children and if the children identified with *them* using hearing aids. For example, one mother reported that her older child said, "Same, same," pointing to herself and her mother. Hopefully, deaf infants will develop better language skills because their parents used hearing aids.

BINAURAL AMPLIFICATION

Almost all of the children in Infant Center were binaurally aided, except for babies with *no* measurable response in one ear. The study presented by Yonovitz (1974) at the American Speech and Hearing Association Conference reinforced our clinical acceptance of *binaural* amplification. In his study, hearing children were seated in an anechoic chamber with electret microphones placed behind their ears. Yonovitz used the Ross and Lerman (1970) WIPI (Word Intelligibility by Picture Identification) test. Speech stimuli were generated from a loudspeaker directly in front, while from two side speakers placed at $60°$ angles, noise was generated at five signal-to-noise ratios. Recordings from the electret microphones were made and then fed to hearing-impaired children in a monaural versus binaural mode. The binaural mode proved significantly better than the monaural mode.

The binaural array recommended for babies contained aids with similar gain, maximum power output, and frequency response, although we followed Barbara Franklin's (1969) work with interest. She compared the effect on consonant discrimination when a low frequency band was added at various intensities either to an ear receiving a high frequency band or to the *opposite* ear. With normal children, she found a significant increase in discrimination in noise when the low frequency band was added *only* to the *opposite* ear. A follow-up study with pathological ears showed that only consonant intelligibility for plosives and fricatives was improved. Franklin used six subjects with dissimilar audiometric configurations, which limited the impact of her work. Therefore, on a conservative basis, for babies with similar audiometric configurations, we recommended similar electroacoustical systems.

Criteria for Hearing Aid Recommendations

Babies and toddlers were in our program for at least a year or more before hearing aid recommendations were finalized. During this time, aids were loaned and repaired free of charge. A trial period made a difference with some children, but once an aid was decided on, an infant used it for most of the year. Criteria for recommending aids were:

1. Real ear aided pure tone and speech measurements.
2. Trial use of aids with different electroacoustical characteristics.
3. Parental and child acceptance of the aids.
4. Educational observation of the child's responses with the aids. This included response to different vowel sounds /a/, /o/, /e/ at varying distances, response to name, songs, general language, etc., with reports being made weekly by the Infant Center teacher after home visits. Information gleaned from home visits was critical (Rubin, 1976).
5. The development of listening skills and speech and language over an extended period of time.

Extended Low Frequency Amplification

When a baby demonstrated hearing through 4,000 Hz, low frequencies were filtered. This practice was based on the phenomona of upward spread of masking demonstrated by Danaher, Osberger, and Pickett (1973) and by Villchur (1973), who showed that speech discrimination in adults with profound sensorineural hearing loss was impaired at suprathershold levels by low frequencies. Villchur found a release of masking when the lows were compressed at suprathreshold levels and recommended a compression analyzer for hearing aids at the *low* frequencies which could be incorporated into a hearing aid.

NEED FOR INFANT HABILITATION PROGRAM

Hearing evaluation for high risk infants should begin early in life and diagnosis should be made by 3 months of age. New diagnostic techniques are now being developed, such as electrocochleography, cardiac audiology in response to speech signals, brainstem audiology, and other techniques which will reduce the uncertainties of infant hearing loss. Infant habilitation and amplification should not await test developments nor should it be *prolonged* by administrative red tape, reimbursement schedules, and long waiting lists. Intervention within the first few months of life for mother and child has a ripple effect. It influences the acquisition of speech and language, the development of the ego, and generates family stability. The electroacoustic aiding of the baby should have the highest priority in the habilitative program.

LITERATURE CITED

Castle, W. E., and I. Ventry. 1967. Conference on hearing aid evaluation procedures. ASHA Rep. 2: 27–38.

Curlee, R. F. 1975. Manpower resources and needs in speech pathology/ audiology. ASHA Rep. 17(4): 265–273.

Danaher, E. M., M. J. Osberger, and J. M. Pickett. 1973. Discrimination of formant frequency transitions in synthetic vowels. J. Speech & Hearing Res. 16: 439–451.

Ehrlich, C. H., E. Shapiro, B. D. Kimball, and M. Huttner. 1973. Communication skills in five year old children with high risk neonatal histories. J. Speech & Hearing Res. 16: 522–529.

Eimas, P. D. 1974. Linguistic processing of speech by young infants. In R. L. Schiefelbusch and L. L. Lloyd (eds.), Language Perspectives–Acquisition, Retardation and Intervention, pp. 56–73. University Park Press, Baltimore.

Eisenberg, R. B. 1970. The organization of human behavior. J. Speech & Hearing Res. 13: 453–471.

Franklin, B. 1970. The effect on consonant discrimination of combining a low-frequency passband in one ear and a high-frequency passband in the other ear. J. Audit. Res. 9: 365–378.

Franklin, B. 1972. The effect of low frequency band (240–480 Hz.) of speech on consonant discrimination in hearing-impaired subjects. Presented at the ASHA meeting, California, CUNY, New York.

Greenstein, J. 1975. Research in the effectiveness of early intervention on language development. Presented at the Infant Center Workshop, Lexington School for the Deaf, New York.

Jeffers, J., T. Behrens, M. Rubin, S. McDonald, and R. Kasten. 1973. Standards for hearing aids. J. Acad. Rehab. Audiol. 6: 1.

Porter, T. 1974. Otoadmittance measurements. Amer. Ann. Deaf. 119(1): 47–52.

Ross, M., and J. Lerman. 1970. A picture identification test for hearing children. J. Speech & Hearing Res. 13: 44–53.

Rubin, M. T., M. H. Rubin, and T. Jupiter. 1975. Audiological assessment of deaf infants and their deaf parents with a habilitation program designed for the entire family. Presented at the ASHA meeting, Washington, D. C., Lexington School for the Deaf, New York.

Rubin, M. T. 1976. Amplification for infants and young children. In Audiology, A Continuing Journal of Education. Vol. 1, No. 2. Grune & Stratton, Inc., New York.

Villchur, E. 1973. Signal processing to improve speech intelligibility in perceptive deafness. J. Acoust. Soc. 53: 1,646–1,655.

Yonovitz, A. 1974. Binaural intelligibility. Presented at the ASHA meeting, Nevada, Speech and Hearing Institute, Texas Medical Center, Houston, Texas.

HEARING AID EVALUATION PROCEDURES WITH CHILDREN

Jane R. Madell

In the last 4 or 5 years, as people have become more aware that audiologists can and do tests very young children, the average age of identification of hearing-impaired children has decreased. The decrease in age of identification and the earlier use of hearing aids resulted in a change in hearing aid evaluation procedures.

TRIAL USE OF AMPLIFICATION

Experience has shown that it is essential to provide every child with a period of adjustment to amplification before attempting to make a decision about which hearing aid is best for a child. Different children respond differently to amplification, and the best audiometric procedures may not provide enough information about choosing hearing aids until it is known how a particular child will respond with a hearing aid. The amount of time a child needs to adjust to amplification is variable and not dependent solely on the degree of hearing loss. Clearly, a child who has a moderate or moderately severe hearing loss will take less time to adjust to amplification than a child with a profound hearing loss, but there is variability within each category of hearing loss. Experience shows that a very young child with a moderate hearing loss may need 2 to 3 months to adjust to amplification until a reliable hearing aid evaluation can be performed. A child with a profound hearing loss may take as long as 6 to 8 months on trial amplification before a good judgment about the hearing aid can be made. Rather than make a recommendation quickly which may later be regretted, the audiologist should make a temporary judgment after the audiometric evaluation and choose a hearing aid to lend to the child. Then the parents, the clinician, and the audiologist follow the child at regular intervals and make some valid judgments about how the child is responding. During the period of trial amplification, hearing aids may be changed several times until the child demonstrates the use of residual hearing to the best advantage. Once it is judged that the child has adjusted to amplification, a serious hearing aid evaluation procedure can begin.

HEARING AID EVALUATING PROCEDURES

Need for Impedance Testing

Impedance testing should precede every hearing aid evaluation session. Often a child may not be responding well with his or her hearing aids, and the next day the child wakes up with a bad cold. Had impedance testing been done, that result might have been predicted.

Evaluation as an Ongoing Procedure

A hearing aid evaluation on a young child cannot be completed at one sitting. For some children, only one aid can be tested before the child ceases to respond well. For others, three hearing aids can be tried. Therefore, a hearing aid evaluation is an ongoing procedure which may take time. Of course, completion of the evaluation in as short a time as possible is desirable, but not at the expense of failing to find the best hearing aid for the child.

Use of Speech Stimuli

Clearly the goal of the hearing aid evaluation is to insure that the child can use his residual hearing for understanding speech. With that goal in mind, it is not sufficient to obtain responses to pure tone stimuli or narrow band noise stimuli in evaluating hearing aids. Since the concern is speech reception, the child's ability to respond to speech stimuli should be regarded as the critical element of the hearing aid evaluation.

Use of W-22 Speech Tests and WIPI Test

Our hearing aid evaluation is usually begun by obtaining thresholds for warbled pure tones or narrow band noise stimuli. Then a speech awareness threshold is obtained. Every attempt is made to get as much speech information as possible since speech perception and reception is the goal of the use of the hearing aid. As a child becomes older and has been in speech, hearing, and language therapy, the child develops the ability to make some auditory discriminations. A great deal of effort is expended to discover which stimuli the child can discriminate using his listening skills alone. These stimuli are used in the hearing aid evaluation. Our procedure will vary depending on the child, the hearing loss, and the child's auditory skills, but an attempt is made to evaluate speech discrimination with *every* child who has any speech discrimination ability whatsoever. The goal in speech discrimination testing is to be able to use the Central Institute for the Deaf's (CID) W-22 word list. However, nonstandard speech discrimination techniques are used with younger children. For example, if the child is able to discriminate three words through audition, then a threshold for those three words is obtained. This threshold does not represent a standard speech reception threshold, but it yields valuable information. Using this technique, children may demonstrate speech reception thresholds which are 10 or 15 dB better for one hearing aid than for another although the pure tone thresholds obtained with both hearing aids are the same. Just 10 or 15 dB can make a big difference when the child is attempting to discriminate speech in a nontest situation. As the child's abilities improve, more standard techniques are used. The WIPI test by Ross and Lerman is used on a regular basis and has been a very useful test. The CID W-22 lists and PBK lists are also used regularly. The CID PBK lists, the WIPI, and the nonstandardized informal speech tests are used only when the child cannot perform on the W-22 list. A score of 28% on the W-22 yields more useful information for the audiologist than can be elicited from the WIPI or nonstandard test score. Knowing what sounds a child can and cannot discriminate helps determine what kind of auditory training he needs.

Development of Speech Discrimination Abilities

We have a high level of expectation for children. By the time he or she is in the third grade, a child with a 70-dB hearing loss should have a speech discrimination score on a standard W-22 test of about 70% without the use of visual cues. It is expected that a child of the same age who has a 95- or 100-dB hearing loss will have a discrimination score between 20 and 40% on a standard W-22 without the use of visual cues. By evaluating the child's speech discrimination ability using both standard and nonstandard techniques, the audiologist is able to provide some information to both the family and the clinician about how well the child is using his or her residual hearing.

MONAURAL VERSUS BINAURAL AMPLIFICATION

There are other factors to consider in choosing a hearing aid—such as the decision between monaural and binaural amplification. The arguments in favor of each are well known. There are a number of children (more than many of us would have thought) who perform significantly better with monaural amplification than with binaural amplification. Decisions need to be individualized so that children are not fitted binaurally who really perform better monaurally. This can be done in several ways.

When a child first gets a hearing aid, two earmolds are made, and the aid is alternated between ears for a few weeks so that the clinician and the audiologist can make a judgment about whether the child appears to be functioning better with the hearing aid in one ear than in the other. Then the child is tested with amplification monaurally, in each ear alternately, and binaurally. The same routine is followed in the therapy situation. The literature supports these procedures. In 1930, Katz and Salis evaluated hearing-impaired people and obtained PB max curves unilaterally and bilaterally. They discovered that there was a sizeable population that did considerably better unilaterally. We have found this same result. Some older children reported that they are unhappy with two aids and that they hear better with one aid. This happens sometimes after several years of wearing binaural amplification. Thus, great care must be taken to assure the child the best auditory environment during the early years, a time so very important for the development of auditory skills.

EAR-LEVEL VERSUS BODY-WORN AMPLIFICATION

Another major decision centers around the choice of ear-level versus body-worn hearing aids. For numerous reasons, ear-level aids are preferred for every child. Fortunately, ear-level hearing aids have improved greatly in the last few years. However, experience with older children has led to a change in thinking about the younger ones. Many older children who are 9 or 10 years of age demonstrate the kind of speech discrimination scores discussed earlier. These children were able to express verbally what they were receiving auditorily with different hearing aids. Initially, many of these youngsters said that they did not want to wear body aids and they asked for an ear-level hearing aid. That request is familiar to any audiologist who works with children.

A hearing aid evaluation was begun with ear-level hearing aids having the same electroacoustic characteristics as the body aid with which the child had performed well. In several cases, the child reported that the ear-level hearing aid was not as good as his own body aid, and speech discrimination test scores bear this out. In therapy both the child and the clinician said that the aid was not good enough. It is difficult to explain why this happened, but there appear to be children whose functioning may be significantly better with a body aid than with an ear-level hearing aid. Recently several manufacturers made up powerful ear-level hearing aids with external receivers, which has made it possible for many children to use ear-level aids satisfactorily.

Maximum Power Output for Children

A third major concern is the maximum power output setting for hearing aids. A child should be exposed to no more than 120- or 125-dB maximum power output (MPO). It was a matter of great concern in 1974 that a large hearing aid manufacturer took one of its very powerful body aids whose MPO was 144 dB and put a microphone-telephone switch on the hearing aid at the request of some schools for the deaf who wanted children to use that hearing aid in a loop system. The thought of numerous children wearing hearing aids with a MPO of 144 dB is very frightening because exposure to that level of noise for a period of time may cause threshold shifts. Deaf children cannot afford to lose any of their residual hearing. Output must carefully be limited. Each child must be evaluated to determine what maximum output that particular child can tolerate, and the child should not be allowed to use more than he or she can tolerate. This is the only way to be certain that a child will not have further deterioration as the result of overamplification.

Vibrotactile Aids for Children with Corner Audiograms

In the past 3 or 4 years, a population of deaf children has presented a real dilemma. These are a group of children who have no measurable hearing unaided and who demonstrate thresholds of 80 and 90 dB wearing a hearing aid that has a MPO of 140 dB. One of these children is a rubella child, two of the children have hereditary hearing loss, and the other four have unknown etiology. Their degree of hearing loss clearly presents a major problem. One of the procedures used with this population was to fit the children binaurally with one air-conduction hearing aid and a second hearing aid worn as a bone-conduction aid. The child wore the bone-conduction hearing aid either on the wrist or taped to any bone that was easily accessible. It provided a vibrotactile stimulus. This seemed to be working minimally well. Children who had no measurable hearing increased the amount of babbling somewhat while using vibrotactile stimuli.

FINAL STEPS IN HEARING AID EVALUATION

The last part of the hearing aid evaluation begins once a child can do well with a particular hearing aid or aids. The child is loaned that hearing aid or aids for a week or two during which time the clinician, the parents, and the audiologist are asked to evaluate how the child functions with the amplification. At what distance can he or she hear you call his name? Can he or she follow commands at 2 feet and 4 feet? Have there been changes in the amount of vocalization, type of vocalization, quality of the vocalization? These judgments are recorded. Then another aid is tried and aids are changed until the audiologist is satisfied that the child is functioning as well as he or she is able to function. Then the child wears the recommended hearing aids for a couple of weeks to see if the expectations turned out to be correct.

Trial Period

Sometimes, before purchase of the aid, the child is not doing as well as was expected during the hearing aid evaluation. There may have been a change in hearing itself, which is very common with very young children. There may have been a clinical error in judgment. Sometimes the child is just beginning to use the telephone or to listen on the telephone and, although the child may be doing very well in the classroom situation with the new aid, he or she may be doing terribly on the telephone. The family may feel that telephone use is very important for this child and so the hearing aids have to be reevaluated and another decision made. By giving the trial period immediately before purchase, correction of an error is allowed.

SUMMARY

Hearing aid evaluation procedures, including extensive trials, may sound like a long, drawn-out program. While it is desirable to do hearing aid evaluations quickly, experience has demonstrated that, if a child is to develop the best use of his or her residual hearing, this amount of effort must be expended in order to be certain that the best possible hearing aid for each and every child has been recommended.

LITERATURE CITED

Katz, F. G., and G. V. Salis. 1930. Quantitative Hörprufüng mit Sprache. Ztschr. Hals-Nasen Ohrenheilkunde 26: 106–126.

HEARING AIDS FOR INFANTS AND CHILDREN: NONINSTRUMENTAL SELECTION CRITERIA

Annette Zaner

WHAT ARE NONINSTRUMENTAL CRITERIA?

Noninstrumental criteria are those criteria in hearing aid evaluations that are not related to the electroacoustic properties of particular hearing aids or to the patient's audiological status. Nor are they related to any psychoacoustic measurements obtained with different aids. In hearing aid evaluations for adults or older children, noninstrumental criteria are those considered in the category, "subject's choice," or "subjective preference." With preschool children, the noninstrumental criteria are those considered by parents, teachers, or clinicians working with the children in language stimulation programs, when those observers "report" on the child's comparative performance (or behavior) when wearing different aids. Noninstrumental criteria are an integral part of the *loaner* model for hearing aid evaluations with preschool children.

At the Mount Carmel Guild (and this procedure is similar at other centers where diagnostic and rehabilitative audiology is practiced), reliance on noninstrumental criteria is apparently inversely related to the age of the patient undergoing a hearing aid evaluation. That is, although subjective, qualitative reactions may be elicited routinely from adults and older children, such input constitutes only a small part of the total evaluation. Conversely, with preschool children for whom loaner aids are a routine part of the hearing aid selection procedure, the final decision about which of several presumably either comparable or selectively variant aids is the best is heavily dependent upon the use of noninstrumental criteria.

"Loaner" Hearing Aid Programs Delay Language Acquisition

One area of clear agreement among different professionals is the philosophical notion that the earlier the identification and provision of appropriately managed amplification, the better the chance for the child to realize near potential in language development. It is this audiologist's contention, however, that the *loaner* program model used with preschool children, wherein ratings gleaned from noninstrumental criteria are given great credence, works in direct contradiction to that philosophy. That is, by accepting as valid the use of noninstrumental criteria in selecting appropriate amplification for preschool children, the result helps to delay the language acquisition and development process.

WHAT IS THE LOANER MODEL?

The *loaner* model is that method of hearing aid selection in which three or four aids are chosen as appropriate amplification, and then each aid is loaned to the child, in succession, for periods of approximately 1 month each. Various noninstrumental criteria are employed to help determine which of the several aids is the "best" one for the child, and then that aid is recommended for purchase. These criteria, reported on by parents, clinicians, and/or teachers, include: response to voice, response to various environmental sounds, visual contact, behavioral changes (including reactions to the instrument itself), localization, vocal and verbal repetitions, reactions to isolated phonemic utterances, auditory comprehension, etc.

How Does It Work?

This procedure of loaning aids to preschool children for periods of time in order to help determine which one of several is *the* best aid is an attempt to replicate the adult hearing aid evaluation model. When conducting hearing aid evaluations with adults, it is recommended procedure that certain speech tests be used in evaluating the patient's aided performance. The ASHA *Conference on Hearing Aid Procedures* (1967) reported on the necessity for running these tests with several aids. It is essential to include a number of different aids because, although "Hearing aids may have similar gain, output, and frequency-response characteristics, . . . (they still may) . . . differ considerably in distortion and other unidentified parameters which can adversely affect hearing performance."

With preschool children, the adult model is not applicable because of the inability to use standardized tests of speech discrimination. Theoretically, then, the *loaner* procedures represent a modification of the adult hearing aid evaluation procedures, employing noninstrumental criteria for the purpose of comparing hearing performance with different aids.

Why Is a Loaner Program Commonly Used?

Noninstrumental criteria are widely relied upon. Northern and Downs (1974) give an excellent, detailed description of hearing aid selection procedures for nonverbal preschoolers. "This procedure," they suggest, "should allow a selection of one or two acceptable aids which can be recommended. If there is any question," they continue, "a trial of the finally selected aids can be suggested. During the trials, observations of the child's performance with each aid can be made by parents, teachers, or clinicians. From these observations the ultimate selection can be made."

In describing the hearing aid evaluation of a child who was approximately 3 years of age when the audiogram was completed, Miller and Polisar (1964) report that, "Four . . . aids were loaned . . . for a period of one month each and the parents were given training in helping the child use . . . aids at home and in observing the child's responses to amplification under different conditions. Reports of . . . responses . . . were made by the parents . . . to enable clinicians to reach final decision." In another case history, the authors report that "a series of . . . aids have been loaned to the family, and the child's responses . . . observed carefully by the parents and reported to the hearing therapist."

Sanders (1971) suggests that ". . . the successful selection and adjustment of hearing aids for young children must depend not only on careful evaluations of clinical test results, but also upon observations made during a trial period of auditory training. . . . His responses during this period are more likely to be accurate indicators of the benefit . . . he derives . . . than any information . . . (obtained) . . . in a formal clinical setting."

And, finally, "ASHA Reports" (1967), although it does not specifically mention a *loaner* procedure with very young preschoolers, in effect supports the use of noninstrumental criteria when it recommends a period of "prognostic therapy," which service ". . . provides for the trial use of alternative aids, molds, and settings, as well as training." During these trials the child's reaction is watched, ". . . both momentarily and from one activity to another . . . ," and the child is . . . "under observation during feeding, playing and sleeping."

HOW DOES ACCEPTANCE OF NONINSTRUMENTAL
CRITERIA IN HEARING AID SELECTION
CONTRADICT EARLY AMPLIFICATION PHILOSOPHY?

It is the unquestionalbe good intention of all involved with preschool hearing-impaired children to provide amplification as early as possible and to do as much as possible to insure that the amplification provided is the best available. However, having ascertained the child's electroacoustic amplification requirements, a 2- to 4- (and often stretched to 6-) month *loaner* period can be a serious waste of time at a critical period in the child's language development. Because aids of similar electroacoustic characteristics can have "... distortion and other parameters which can adversely affect hearing performance" (ASHA Reports, 1967), the use of several different aids is recommended when doing hearing aid evaluations with adults, wherein the adult's hearing performance with the different aids is compared, when standardized speech tests are administered.

Substituting noninstrumental criteria for standardized speech tests as a modification of the recommended adult hearing aid evaluation procedures, for preschool children, has highly questionable validity. With an adult, the premise is that an adventitious loss of hearing leaves the patient with an intact linguistic system that can be utilized in the test situation. Theoretically, the amplification instrument which has the least distortion or other detrimental qualities will enable the patient to demonstrate best hearing performance. That aid, then, can be recommended as the best one for that patient. Acceptance of reports from adults in the preschool child's environment on how much better a child may localize, respond to a doorbell, mimic the teacher's words, or recognize a dog's bark with one aid as compared to others over a period of several months cannot be compared to the assessment of adult linguistic hearing performance with different aids in one sitting.

Loaner Program Disadvantages

First, the child with a congenital hearing impairment is going to learn language through a distorted system. To insist that it can be scientifically determined which amplification system has the least distortion for that child through observation of responses to nonlinguistic auditory stimuli is pretentious.

Second, the preschool child going through the typical *loaner* aid process is in that maturational phase when normally hearing children experience rapid growth in language development. Modern psycholinguistic theory posits that hearing-impaired children have an innate capacity for language acquisition comparable to that of their normally hearing peers. It can be expected, then, that rapid changes will occur in youngsters' abilities to use amplification for language acquisition during this period, especially if they are enrolled in language stimulation programs. To assume that the use of noninstrumental criteria with different hearing aids issued over a 2- to 4- or 6-month period can net meaningful data on comparative linguistic performance of preschool hearing-impaired children is not appropriate.

Even if it could be assumed that the aid with the least detrimental distortion for that child could be determined from the preschool patient's comparative behaviors, there is no way of guaranteeing that the *observation* of that behavior is consistent, reliable, repeatable, or valid. Those observations are dependent upon essentially untrained, often emotionally biased, third parties for reporting on noninstrumental criteria, and yet reports are the basis for final decisions in selecting hearings aids for preschool children.

Many years ago, during hearing aid evaluations performed for groups of severely hearing-impaired preteen and teenaged children from a school for the deaf, the youngsters were asked which aid *they* liked best. Before everyone dashed out to buy stock in the favorite company, several of the particularly verbal children were asked, "Why?" Their consistent answer was, "Because it's gold." And, no matter how remotely the instruments were situated—on a baffle board, behind the patient, for instance—they always knew the one they wanted, perhaps by touching the receiver, or noting the thickness of the cord, and their choices were almost never ascribed to relative appreciation of acoustic stimuli.

It is the contention in this paper that dependence on noninstrumental criteria for final decisions in hearing aid selection for preschoolers is an invalid and time-wasting procedure. The *loaner* program, with its reliance on noninstrumental selection criteria, hinders important work of language stimulation and general habilitation. Experience has shown that, when the final decision about an aid is dependent upon comparative reports, using noninstrumental criteria, even though the child may simultaneously be enrolled in a preschool program and receiving training with amplification, everyone seems to be waiting for the pronouncement about which aid is "the" aid for that child, before making the necessary commitment to the reality of the child wearing his or her own aid. Parents, teachers, clinicians, and audiologists divert undo amounts of their time and energy from language training into fitting, changing, refitting, and manipulating different comparable aids on the child, and then watching for responses which in the end may or may not be related to differences in the amplification systems.

WHY DO AUDIOLOGISTS WORKING WITH PRESCHOOL CHILDREN CONTINUE TO RELY UPON NONINSTRUMENTAL CRITERIA FOR FINAL DECISIONS IN HEARING AID SELECTION?

Several interrelated factors contribute to the continued inappropriate use of noninstrumental selection criteria. First, perhaps because clinical audiology still is almost entirely dependent upon behavioral measures for threshold determinations, perhaps because commercially available electronic amplification is not yet highly perfected, and perhaps because there are still uncertainties about as yet undetermined, potentially measurable parameters of hearing as they relate to perception and comprehension of speech, audiologists are generally insecure about their audiometric findings in preschool children and are, therefore, reluctant to make decisions on amplification solely on the basis of those audiograms plus the use of available electroacoustic criteria.

Use of Adult Model for Selecting an Aid

Second, when engaged in hearing aid evaluations with preschool children, audiologists seem inextricably locked into the adult model, with its recommended comparisons of hearing performance with several different aids. The purpose behind that comparison procedure is to determine which of several appropriate aids enables the patient to demonstrate best hearing performance. The underlying premise is, that with continued persistence, "the" appropriate aid will be found for that patient. This system is somewhat reminiscent of optometric procedures, wherein the optometrist, having refracted the patient's eyes and making a gross correction, then asks the patient to participate with him in the finer correction, by the "Which do you like best?" process. Unfortunately, the adjustments that can be made on hearing aids do not compare with those possible for lenses, and the "distortion" factor is not directly measureable. Furthermore, it was demonstrated by Miller and Sprung (1956), that when patients were retested with the aids that yielded the "best" and the "worst" results, the original findings were not upheld. It seems clear, then, that there is not yet "one" appropriate aid for a particular hearing-impaired individual.

Adult Model Myth is Perpetuated in Textbooks

A third factor that contributes to the continued use of noninstrumental criteria is the promulgation of this practice in texts dealing with both clinical and rehabilitative audiology. The procedure is taught in the training institution, practiced in early work experience, and then reinforced as still appropriate in continued education.

HOW SHOULD AUDIOLOGISTS SELECT APPROPRIATE AMPLIFICATION FOR PRESCHOOL CHILDREN?

Of the major problems currently faced by audiology, the insecurity experienced in obtaining valid pure tone audiograms with preschool children appears outstanding. This insecurity may be related to negative propagandizing by pediatricians and other medical specialists who continue to counsel parents to "wait until the child is old enough to be tested." It may be caused by the difficulty such testing may present to inexperienced audiologists or to individuals who work as the only audiologist in a clinical setting. It may be caused by the audiologist's general lack of familiarity with principles of child development, or it may be generated by the institutionalized sexist myth that says that only "special," "motherly" types of clinicians are able to get reliable results from preschoolers. Whichever of these factors is operative, the field of audiology must deal with this insecurity and find a means of enabling trained audiologists to be better prepared to test preschoolers (a sizeable proportion of all of our caseloads), and then to feel confident about their results. Those audiologists who routinely examine many preschoolers, including those who are multiply handicapped, continue to report success in their testing procedures and in follow-up. Intertest reliability is high.

NEED FOR VALID AUDIOLOGICAL TESTING

With added confidence in audiological work-ups, which ought routinely to include acoustic reflex testing, audiologists should be able to eliminate time-consuming, nonproductive dependence upon noninstrumental criteria in hearing aid selection procedures for preschool children. With secure reliance on audiometric data and careful consideration of the required and available electroacoustic properties, a firm decision can be made about a hearing aid earlier than is done when noninstrumental criteria are used for final judgments. Select the aid, expedite its purchase, and get on with the job of training parent, teacher, and child to use it.

ADDITIONAL NEGATIVE SIDE-EFFECTS OF DEPENDING ON NONINSTRUMENTAL CRITERIA

The use of noninstrumental criteria for final decisions necessitates obtaining and maintaining a large stock of *loaner* aids that are always in excellent repair. Unless the institution housing the program has sufficient funds to purchase such a stock and keep it in good working order, the need for the *loaner* aid stock places that institution (and often its audiologists) in a position of dependence on various manufacturers, distributors, or individual hearing aid vendors. Especially when the audiology profession is struggling for "independence" (if not "survival"), it is well to reexamine the dependency that has been created in relation to the questionable benefits a *loaner* program nets.

Audiologists are a knowledgeable group of professionals, with much to offer hearing-impaired children and their families in diagnostic and rehabilitative audiological expertise. It is hoped that as they feel more confident about their findings, they will need to rely less on noninstrumental criteria in conducting hearing aid evaluations for preschool children.

LITERATURE CITED

American Speech and Hearing Association (ASHA). 1967. Conference on hearing aid evaluation procedures. Reports No. 2: 28–41.

Miller, M. H. 1972. Hearing Aids. Bobbs-Merrill Company, Inc., New York.

Miller, M. H., and I. A. Polisar. 1964. Audiological Evaluation of the Pediatric Patient, pp. 74–77. Charles C Thomas, Publisher, Springfield, Ill.

Miller, M. H., and A. J. Sprung. 1956. Variability of discrimination scores in clinical hearing aid selection. Presented at the American Speech and Hearing Association meeting, Chicago.

Northern, J. L., and M. P. Downs. 1974. Hearing in Children, p. 235. The Williams & Wilkins Company, Baltimore.

Sanders, D. A. 1971. Aural Rehabilitation, p. 162. Prentice-Hall, Inc., Englewood Cliffs, N. J.

COGNITION IN THE DEVELOPMENT OF LISTENING SKILLS

Leahea F. Grammatico

The development of listening skills and the development of thinking skills are two critical issues facing teachers who are preparing children to become fully integrated into our rapidly changing society. The development of these two skills cannot be separated because cognitively based tasks that motivate the child to think form the content for listening. The inevitable outgrowths of these interrelated tasks are language and speech provided that hearing-impaired children have acquired consistent, continuous, and appropriately selected amplification.

COGNITIVE APPROACH

Systematically defined and developed strategies that capitalize on the child's state of intellectual development, as defined by Jean Piaget, are the challenge facing teachers today. Even a very young child acquires information from a variety of sources—the adults with whom he interacts, the children with whom he plays, picture books and magazines, television, toys, household routines, pets, foods, his own changing body with varying clothing needs, sand, dirt, water, observation of worms crawling, butterflies flying—an endless variety of experiences that are foundational for language development and consequent expansion.

Hierarchy of Teacher's Questions

The cognitive approach for content-based material is a process that is used by the teacher in this fashion. First, she presents the object by holding it under her mouth. The question always asked, which the teacher herself

117

answers, is: "What do you see?" For example, a toothbrush would be presented in the following manner:

Teacher: "What do you see? A toothbrush. This is a toothbrush." The teacher then provides a model of how the object is used.

Teacher: "What do you see? A toothbrush. This is a toothbrush." The teacher then provides a model of how the object is used.
Teacher: "You brush your teeth with a toothbrush."

Later the questions will be expanded to:

"What do you know about ———————————?"
"How are these two things alike?"
"What would happen if?"

Much later, when similarities have been established, the question: "How are they different?" would be asked.

This sequence of questions is very important—even critical. It enables the child to organize what he knows so that the teacher can expand and, thus, increase knowledge, stimulate thinking, and expand language and speech skills. Too many teachers make teaching a *telling* activity rather than using questions to allow the child to express what he knows.

Illustrative Lesson—Telling Activity

The first step *is* a telling activity. Language must be poured in before one can expect to get it back. Language is the *content* for listening.

For example, you may place three large pictures such as a car, a toothbrush, and a cup on the chalk ledge of a flannel board. Standing behind the child you would say:

"You come to school in the car."
"You brush your teeth with a toothbrush. Toothbrush."
"You drink out of a cup."

If the child fails to identify the correct picture, you would put the picture under your mouth as the child watches and say:

"Toothbrush. You brush your teeth with a toothbrush.
Now listen."

Behind the child's back, repeat the exact sentence again.

A more difficult task is to draw a known object on the board such as a toothbrush. Standing behind the child you would say:

"If that's a toothbrush, what's missing?"

Children readily draw in the toothpaste as a line on the bristles, although they don't know the name for toothpaste. This exercise becomes more difficult as you add an apple tree with missing apples, a comb with missing teeth, and a tricycle with a missing wheel.

No child can live even 1 year without acquiring many ideas about his action-oriented world. He will convey these ideas if he is encouraged to do so. I have yet to see a group of little children who didn't have lots of bruises that are all usually acquired in different ways. If you bruise your leg falling off a tricycle, it's important to compare your bruise with the ones acquired by the other members of the group. After all, "*my* bruise may be bigger than yours!" "I'm *sure* it hurt more!"

Teaching Strategies

Those who are involved in the management of children have a wealth of information at their disposal. They know, for example, that the phrase and later the sentence is the unit of language. Too often they forget this. Little children are always bringing bags of "stuff" to share (if they are hearing children), "news" if they are deaf. Very often the conversation goes something like this:

Teacher: "Do you have something to show us?"
Child: "Yes," or maybe only a nod of the head.
Teacher: "How many do you have? What color is it or them? Where did you get it or them? What do you do with it or them? How much did it cost?"

These are a wealth of questions requiring usually one word responses. Even the questions are not always in the correct syntactical order. "What color is it?" may precede "How many?" and nobody says, "Yellow, three balls."

I always wonder when I hear this kind of exercise just who is practicing language! Naming colors, objects, numbers, and days of the week will never prepare children to talk about astronauts or computers, even with consistent, continuous, and appropriately selected amplification.

A child with enough language to answer the above questions should be asked to *describe* what he has brought to share. If a child does not have the language to answer the above questions, the teacher should supply *all* of the information. For example, the teacher might say:

"David brought something to show us. David, let me peek. I see a toy dog. David brought his dog to show us. Look!"

Produce the dog and say:

"David brought his dog to show us. Dogs bark. Puppies say *erf, erf.* Big dogs say *woof, woof.*"

Teacher: David, can you say, I brought?	*Child*:	"I brought."
Teacher: "my dog."	*Child*:	"my dog."
Teacher: "I brought my dog."	*Child*:	"I brought my dog."

Teacher: "*You* brought *your* dog. He looks like a friendly dog."

Expansion of Listening Skills

A simple melody using "Eyes, nose, mouth, tongue, one, two, three, four, five" will expand vocabulary, make learning fun and motivate the child to think. Unless "listening" or if one prefers, "auditory training," is systematically developed to enable the child to process information, it is a waste of his time and the teacher's. In terms of listening skills, it is much easier to listen to large segments of information than very small ones. As one of my young moppets carefully explained, "I can hear 'electricity' better than I can hear 'it' but I can say 'it' better than I can say 'electricity'." Knowing this, why are deaf children encouraged to express unhappiness with the word "sad"? It's not very specific, can hardly be heard, is difficult to lipread, and isn't nearly as descriptive or contain nearly as much auditory information as the words "frustrated," "depressed," "furious," "unhappy," "angry," or "miserable."

Use of Songs and Music

It's much easier to discriminate two childlike songs than it is to discriminate two sounds. Songs contain a great deal of auditory information. Sounds contain almost no auditory information. The parents of a hearing child do not talk to that child in terms of pure tones or spondaic words—"football," "baseball," "hot dog," or "playground." They sing to their babies. They tell their babies stories. They talk to their babies in sentences. The child's spontaneous speech (which becomes language) begins as verbal utterances that develop into sounds. "Ma, ma, ma, ma" becomes "Mama." Mama expands into "Mama go bye bye." This expands into "Mama, I want more milk." Sentences are expanded into finger plays and songs as the child grows.

Young deaf children develop speech and language in exactly the same way as hearing children do, providing they have been provided with the above described teaching strategies and appropriate amplification which is worn consistently and continuously.

Development of Intonation (Voice Color)

Localization of sound, auditory memory, intonational patterns, and voice color are other interrelated parameters of the development of listening skills and are part of the child's educational experiences all day, every day. If I call one child from a group of flve, I expect only the one I called to turn to me. The development of auditory memory or remembering what has been said is a continuous, ongoing, educational process, especially for the child born with little residual hearing. Teaching the child to raise and lower his voice to develop voice color is of the utmost importance. If someone telephones me and I answer with a lilting "Hi," I've said something quite different than if I respond with a *flat* "Hi."

CHILD-BASED COGNITIVE STRATEGIES

After the child becomes aware of spoken language through stimulus and response activities and has begun to discriminate auditory information, cognitive-based tasks form the content for listening skill activities. The development of cognition or the ability to think is nothing more than teaching a child to organize and reorganize the material he has acquired from a variety of sources.

A teacher must never impose her cognitive scheme on the child. For example, if the words "pig," "dog," "cow," and "giraffe" were written on the board and an adult were asked which one did not belong, an adult would probably say "giraffe" because it's a wild animal and the other three are domestic animals. When this task was presented to a group of 5 and 6-year-old deaf children, one said that the dog didn't belong because it was the "only one that barked." Another said that the pig didn't belong because it was the "only one that gave us bacon." Another said that the cow didn't belong because it was the "only one that gave us milk." Another said that the giraffe didn't belong because it was the "only one with a long neck." These were well-thought-out answers which clearly indicated that only one child was ready for subsuming tasks.

The job of the teacher is to plan teaching-learning experiences that are systematically and hierarchically arranged and to always remember that the fastest way for the young child to acquire information is through hearing.

DISCUSSION

DURABILITY OF CHILDREN'S HEARING AIDS

DR. RUBIN: Should the federal government require industry to build hearing aids for children to last 5 years? It has been estimated that aids currently last about 3 years.

MRS. GRAMMATICO: We hope that there will be some major improvements within the next 5 years in hearing aids and, if so, I would want children to have them. So far, there has not been any change in receivers for 20 years. It took us a long time to get the electret mike and the ceramic mike available in a small package. I want ongoing changes in the hearing aid industry. I do not quite understand why they can't get parts together that would give us better amplification and appropriate amplification in the high frequencies. If hearing aids will be required to last 5 years, it seems to me that the industry will be further toned down. If I could keep people happy for 5 years, I'd expect to become chairman of the board! The commercial person's goal is to make money, right? We have to look at this. I'm not satisfied that the hearing aids we have now should last 5 years. I'd like to see them out 2 weeks from now so we could all get new ones.

In my school, our children have at least three hearing aids, and some have four. We are a very poor private school. There are lots of things in private education you learn to do without. My teachers learn almost immediately that what is needed to teach a child is creativity, a piece of chalk, a chalk board, and a child. We do not, however, skimp on amplification. If a child is on selective slopes of amplification curves and his hearing aid is not working for any reason, we must have a ready loaner available. Our children have to have three or four aids depending on how they are fitted. How do we get the money for this? We go out and give fund-raising speeches. We always take a videotape of the child! Sometimes, we take the child. We write grants. We participate in research areas with the State Department so that our children will get hearing aids. When there is a new hearing aid available that's better than the one that they have had, we change. We do not accept 23 models of hearing aids because they do not have at least 60 dB of gain at 4,000 Hz. There is a new aid with a top mike and some of our children have developed more effective listening skills with that change. Some hearing aids, as far as I am concerned, are outdated. We are not repairing them any more. If consistent and continuous amplification is the goal, we need the tools with which to make this goal possible.

SWITCHING HEARING AIDS

DR. MADELL: I agree that hearing aids have to be changed as often as is indicated. Once a child develops speech discrimination, for example, a new hearing aid may improve that child's speech discrimination. Although binaural hearing aids were purchased last year, we may have to recommend *new* binaural hearing aids this year because the child performs significantly better with the new ones. However, that does not necessarily mean that the old hearing aids have to go into the trash.

Hearing aids should be built to last at least 5 years, but that doesn't mean the same person has to wear them for 5 years. It means that the old hearing aids may be very good for another child after the first child is no longer using them. There are adults who wear their hearing aids for 10 years and children who have worn the same hearing aid for as long as 8 years before having to change aids. This is particularly true of some of the older aids, which somehow lasted longer than the new aids—just as the old cars lasted longer than the new cars. It is possible to make devices which last. Debate is not needed on why they are *not* being made.

DISPOSABLE HEARING AIDS

DR. ZANER: I agree with Jane Madell that the same aid the child has worn for 5 years can continue to be that child's aid except that it may have to be modified. This is an economy that breeds obsolescence. How can we begin to discuss that issue? Should we throw out the car because the ashtrays are dirty? I don't mean it to be a joke. It's a very serious matter. We have to understand that hearing aids are created to be disposed of and to be replaced, in part, at least. That's a very nice goal. The federal

Food and Drug Administration ought to work on *that* goal and a few other things and get a bigger staff!

SPARE HEARING AIDS

DR. RUBIN: Recently some visitors from the Montreal Oral School reported that every child enrolled in that school had two hearing aids and a spare furnished by the government. We asked the principal how that was achieved because in New York State spare hearing aids are *not* issued to children. The principal explained that the government was told it was *absolutely necessary* and, as a result, every child has two aids and a spare.

DR. ZANER: The prices of hearing aids in Canada are somewhat less.

NEED FOR CONSISTENT, FUNCTIONAL AMPLIFICATION

DR. RUBIN: When I visited the Copenhagen schools for the deaf, each classroom had a little parts box—the kind used in an audiology clinic. *Every* child had a spare hearing aid in the parts box neatly labeled with the child's name. If we are really interested in functional amplification— whether we are an oral school or total communication school, or whether we are in a public school or a private school setting—it is equally important for children on Medicaid or on welfare to be issued the same spare hearing aid that a more affluent parent can afford to buy or a more affluent state can afford to provide. In New York City the Bureau for Handicapped Children will not entertain that notion at all. They won't even consider a spare hearing aid. At Lexington, since approximately one-third of our children are registered with the Bureau for Handicapped Children, the school buys spare hearing aids for the children, but that's an inequity. The government spends thousands of dollars to educate children, and it's not reasonable to expect children to learn without consistent, functional amplification.

BINAURAL AMPLIFICATION

MRS. GRAMMATICO: All except three of our children have binaural amplification. One has binaural amplification which will be changed in a couple of weeks. That child is having ear-level hearing aids built for her. Two other children simply do not do as well with binaural amplification as they do with monaural amplification. Hard and fast rules cannot be made about this because the human organism is very complex. General statements are not going to fit all of us.

PROBLEM LEARNERS

MRS. GRAMMATICO: Currently everyone is worrying about what is commonly called "learning disability" or "language disorders." I call these children "problem learners." What is at stake in many cases is teaching disabilities. We have not as yet discovered the strategies for *all* learners.

CROSS AGE GROUPING

MRS. GRAMMATICO: Teachers talk all the time about the fact that their classes of hearing-impaired children have too many levels. They can't get through to them. This is the way life is. Families differ. The children aren't all the same chronologically, but they can all have something to give to that group. An educator uses the strengths in a group of children to their advantage. Children shouldn't be all the same age.

In San Francisco we regroup our children for every activity. If a child is in one group for reading, it doesn't mean that he will be in arithmetic with the same group of children. The group is based on what the children are capable of doing. Who teaches the various subjects depends on the strength of the teacher within that subject area. It's a nontraditional pattern, but it works.

BINAURAL AIDS

DR. MADELL: I agree with Mrs. Grammatico that binaural hearing aids have to be evaluated for every child, but perhaps a disadvantage is created if binaural hearing aids are placed on children before the audiologist finds out whether they are better for that particular child. Many children function better with monaural aids. We have to be cautious in evaluating the situation and not make a priority judgment.

DR. RUBIN: The historical development of the hearing aid may be important in this monaural-binaural controversy. Mark Ross once commented that the reason audiologists always start with monaural aids is that years ago, when hearing aids were developed, they were enormously large. Old-fashioned hearing aids were worn with a carbon pack on the knee and they were big! It would have been almost impossible to use binaural aids under those circumstances. Traditionally, it led to the assumption that monaural aids were the starting point in a hearing aid evaluation.

Our procedure is to start with monaural aids and test each ear. Then we analyze the child's responses—monaural versus binaural. It's the length of testing time that is objectionable in most clinics. It is unilateral deprivation to keep a child on a monaural aid over a long period of time because there are considerable advantages for most children with binaural aids. I am in favor of careful selection and careful audiological assessment, but one need not automatically limit the child to monaural amplification for a long time.

DR. ZANER: I don't believe in fitting monaurally or binaurally until I see the audiological data with the child. No one disagrees with that.

MAXIMUM POWER OUTPUT AND GAIN

DR. ZANER: There have been many statements made about limiting maximum output. I am equally very concerned about gain—about not providing too much gain and thereby overamplifying the child. Audiologists use many different pieces of information to put it all together. The business of just reading audiometric average threshold and making a decision about how much gain should be provided is not enough. Potential recruitment factors are very important in order not to overamplify children.

DR. MADELL: Again it depends on the specific child—especially the learning-disabled child.

DR. ZANER: There appear to be no specific answers about binaural aids for the learning-disabled child, but some of Berlin's research in New Orleans on dicotomous listening skills may provide answers one day. Berlin's experiments have raised many questions about binaural amplification in terms of which is the preferred ear, as well as the relative amplification in each ear when using binaural amplification.

AUDIENCE MEMBER: A number of children that started with monaural hearing aids completely rejected binaural aids at first. After about 1 month's experience with binaural aids they were reevaluated. They responded beautifully and accepted them a lot better. I am convinced that they had been trained to listen with one aid in one ear and the signal was confusing when they were suddenly exposed to two hearing aids.

DR. RUBIN: It takes time to relearn auditory skills even with one new aid. Deaf adults, for example, who have used monaural amplification, have to have a period of learning to assimilate the auditory input when they start to use two aids. At first, there is a slight decrement in a discrimination score which will change after auditory training.

DICHOTIC LISTENING AND EAR DOMINANCE

DR. MADELL: Barbara Franklin applied low frequency amplification to one ear and high frequency amplification to another ear and reported startlingly improved speech discrimination. We tried to replicate her results with body aids and it didn't work. When I reread her original research, I discovered that she used very little gain at a level slightly above threshold, which made a difference. But when the kind of gain that profoundly deaf children need is used, the difference that Franklin reported didn't obtain.

DR. ZANER: What Berlin reported that was so intriguing had to do with the relative gain input (intensity input) to two ears. Following the original Bergman material, fusion is reached when the signal is in the middle of the head. That may be an inappropriate way to use binaural amplification in terms of dicotomous listening. That's one of the exciting, challenging things about Berlin's report. Audiologists may first have to determine which is the dominant ear and then adjust the gain in terms of feeding the higher gain into the appropriate side.

RADIO FREQUENCY AUDITORY
TRAINING UNITS VERSUS PERSONAL HEARING AIDS

DR. RUBIN: At Lexington we use radio frequency auditory trainers in classrooms for older students. Inasmuch as there are no standards for radio frequency auditory trainers, they vary considerably from unit to unit with regard to the amount of gain, the frequency response, and the signal/noise ratio. The signal received in a radio frequency unit is not the same signal received in a child's environmental mike.

We have several criteria for using radio frequency units. The child has to be able to hear himself, his neighbor, and his teacher. The unit should be binaural if possible. It should be a signal that is clear and free from noise. The unit itself should have good fidelity and compression. For very young children who are in open classrooms and are taught on a one-to-one basis, the children use their own hearing aids in order to have a consistent input model. In our intermediate classes, however, there is more class work going on. The children may sit 8 feet from the teacher and radio frequency units bring the teacher's voice close. In a group where some children have very old hearing aids—and haven't had them replaced yet—we can rely on a radio frequency unit and can always provide a spare unit for the child if his radio frequency unit becomes defective. Also, it can be repaired on the spot. It's always working. The teacher's signal can always reach the child wherever he or she is. Therefore, radio frequency group amplification has an advantage for certain age groups who have acquired good speech and language. They need a good teaching model. Of course, the children who use a radio frequency unit are tested audiologically with that unit to see how well they perform compared to their own personal aids.

NEED TO EVALUATE THE TRAINING UNIT

DR. MADELL: This is a question that comes up all the time. All too often children are placed on auditory units without evaluating how they function with the particular unit. It's difficult for a child to have to use three different auditory units in a day, as is required in certain educational settings, and then go home with a hearing aid and have to learn to discriminate speech with four different frequency responses. That's asking a lot of a hearing-impaired child. We forget how difficult that is and request a lot of our children by asking that of them. Even if the child is fortunate enough to use only frequency response, it is incumbent upon audiologists to know how well the child functions with the unit. Too many programs simply put auditory training units on children without evaluating how the children function with the particular unit they are asking them to wear. It may very well be that they function much better with their own hearing aid which they wear all the time.

COST OF HEARING AIDS IN GREAT BRITAIN

AUDIENCE MEMBER: The National Health Service in Scotland is supposed to insure that every child receives at least one hearing aid, possibly two. Most of these hearing aids were originally constructed for adults who were disabled during the war and are not really suitable for children who are born with hearing disabilities. Many schools use one or two of the National Health aids or Medresco aids. More recently, in Britain, there has been tremendous competition commercially, especially from the foreign hearing aids. Schools are saying that they cannot afford to buy these commercial aids. The government will give them National Health aids, but the schools cannot afford these other aids which they feel are probably much better for the children. Recently, in 1974, the government has passed a bill whereby the children are *now* entitled to commercial hearing aids.

DR. RUBIN: What do schools pay for aids in Britain?

AUDIENCE MEMBER: The cost to parents is about £75 for an aid, which is about $200. That's a lot of money. In Britain the cost of living is very different. Schools will be able to be subsidized for getting these aids.

The interesting thing to see in visiting schools around England and Scotland is that some of the kids aren't wearing aids and some are wearing National Health aids, which seems inappropriate. The teachers say, "They won't give us any other aids. We can't get them." Then I go into another school and ask the same question. "Why do you have so many commercial aids in your school? How do you do it?" I'm not talking of London or New York City; I'm talking about provincial places. The head of the school will say to me: "We built up a relationship with our local government, the people who are responsible. We told them we must have these aids. We are convinced that they are crucial to the children's education. We have seen and can demonstrate the potential of the hearing-impaired child. They cannot say to us that we know better than you." In order words, the rapport that has been built up, and the fact that educators are convinced has a large part to play in getting those aids. I don't know if it is substantially different here in smaller communities.

DR. RUBIN: It is a matter of priorities.

HEARING AID TEST EQUIPMENT

DR. ZANER: A lot of equipment is bought because that equipment is manufactured and marketed. To be without it is not to be as updated as the next center. That is something we have to look at very carefully. In a university setting recently I saw incredible amounts of magnificent equipment, which was just sitting there most of the time. In fact, *they* did not need a Brüel and Kjaer hearing aid evaluation box. I might need it in a clinical setting! In that setting, just to show a student what it is seems like an incredible waste of money. A student can go elsewhere to see what it looks like.

Neonatal testing equipment is in the same category. Every pediatrician has to have one. The man on television says that they have to buy it. I don't appreciate that!

DR. RUBIN: In our clinic, one of the most important pieces of equipment that we have is the equipment to analyze hearing aids. I really don't know how we ever did without it—as Jerger once said about an impedance bridge. Very few hospital speech and hearing centers in New York have Brüel and Kjaer equipment.

DR. MADELL: Not all speech and hearing centers need it. Programs that see large numbers of hearing-impaired children who rely heavily on their auditory skills have to have a way to make sure the hearing aids are working. The kids do better when their aids are working. There's only one way to find out if it's working. Holding it up to your ear and listening with a stethoscope is not the right way to do it.

SENSORY AIDS

DR. MADELL: May I describe the sensory aid we are using with deaf children? It is a bone-conduction aid with a body aid which has a very long cord. The body hearing aid has low frequency emphasis because we are looking for vibrotactile responses. Ideally, we would like to use a particular aid because one company has a very large, nice, beautiful bone vibrator.

In the wintertime the children wore it on their wrists. It was kept in place by using a wristband like the one you might use for a sprained wrist. When the weather started to get warm and the kids wanted to wear short sleeved shirts, we ran into a problem. The wires were tangling, especially on the very small kids. We put two-faced tape on the bone vibrator to tape it down. That's probably what will be used next winter also, because it was more comfortable for the child than having a long cord going down his arm.

For auditory training, the vibrator unit is also used. The use of a vibrator with all hearing-impaired children is extremely helpful for pitch, intonation, and inflection (especially for the very profoundly hearing-impaired). The Suvag Auditory Training Units are used for individual speech and auditory training work. That has a very large vibrator that children can wear. With this vibrator on, the children have shown improved inflection and intonation. Vibrators are a very good way to develop many skills that make speech more intelligible.

MONITORING A CHILD'S HEARING AID

DR. RUBIN: How can you monitor an older child to guarantee that his hearing aid is performing at peak efficiency? For example, in Sweden, audiologists collect all the hearing aids in the school every 3 months and run a Brüel and Kjaer acoustic analysis which picks up any deficiency. More frequent acoustic analysis of the aids is certainly in order. On the other hand, a good teacher is very knowledgeable about the child's responses and if, for one reason or another, these are not as optimal as the teacher expects, one can begin to be suspicious that the hearing aid is defective.

CROSS-CHECKING A HEARING AID
WITH BRÜEL AND KJAER EQUIPMENT

MRS. GRAMMATICO: We are underestimating something. There *is* a cross-check on hearing aids. The Brüel and Kjaer equipment performs only as well as its operator. A few months ago at the Hearing and Speech Center, we were getting reports that a particular hearing aid was 100% distorted. According to the Brüel and Kjaer measurement, it was. Actually, we had to have an engineer come out and explain to us what was happening–that the hearing aid had so much low frequency information in its setting that it was not permitting the Brüel and Kjaer to operate correctly. What would someone hear if a hearing aid was 100% distorted? We listened to the hearing aid, and the speech signal was coming through loud and clear. We have a tremendous rapport with the center because we're an affiliated program. We had a big argument. What I heard was, "The Brüel and Kjaer says this." I could listen and know that the Brüel and Kjaer, in this particular instance, was wrong. Another time, the janitor had flipped the switch. Nobody picked that up. These are problems that educators live with.

FONIX EQUIPMENT

MRS. GRAMMATICO: On our school side, we have Fonix equipment. We also do a listening check on the child's hearing aid three times. The mother does the hearing aid check (this is an ongoing parent education program); the classroom teacher does the hearing aid check; and the therapist does the hearing aid check. Every child receives 30 minutes of tutorial instruction per day. If something is radically wrong with the aid, it is checked on the Fonix and then on the Brüel and Kjaer which is available. The audiologist will do it for us. This is valuable information.

There is another check which will tell whether or not a hearing aid is working properly. What about going back to the speech sounds and checking them out? Are you hearing a "k"? Are you hearing a "sh"? One has to learn to listen to the hearing aid. The child's behavior is another indication.

MASTER HEARING AID APPROACH

In our facility we use the working-team approach. In that approach the audiologist evaluates the child clinically and then he sends this information to the educator, who tests the child with a master hearing aid using varying slopes of amplification curves and charts for a 4- to 6-week period to evaluate how the child is doing. Educators use a "Listening Skill" work-sheet. It gives the audiogram at the top, the date, the maximum power output, the slope, the sound pressure level, and the amount of time worked with during that particular day. The content is cognatively based; the outgrowth is speech and language. In other words, the child has a lesson while the teacher records the strategy used and the child's behav-ioral response—what he is doing auditorily. When this is completed, a summary sheet is sent to the audiologist, and the audiologist uses all of this information to make a selection of hearing aids. That's another approach which has been very effective. It makes the educator increasingly aware of the problems in audiology, and the greatest thing is that audiolo-gists have become increasingly aware of what deaf children can do. There is an exchange that was not there 10 years ago.

PARENT RESPONSIBILITIES

DR. MADELL: In our center, audiologists are very careful with very young children's first earmold. The parent is told to get an earmold also, and we ask them to do a listening check of the hearing aid every morning. As the kids get older, audiologists rightfully give parents all the respon-sibility. If there is a normal hearing person in the house, whether it is the parent or another adult, he can listen to the hearing aid every morning. The parents will come and say, "I used to be able to listen to this hearing aid at a three setting, now I can get it up to five." They are right. Something's probably wrong. The batteries may be good, but something is wrong with the hearing aid. An easy check is to try to arrange for a normal hearing person to listen to the aid every day to make sure it's still functioning. If someone listens every day, when the aid stops performing well, the person will be able to recognize the change.

EARMOLD CHECK

DR. RUBIN: We had a very interesting demonstration of that principle. Dr. Dan Ling was demonstrating a speech lesson with a Lexington student, Peter, and the audiologists were aware of Peter's auditory residual when he was aided. Dr. Ling tested Peter at a distance of 5 feet with three vowels: /e/, /a/, and /u/, and Peter did not respond to the vowel /e/. Peter stopped in later to see the audiologist who checked his hearing aid. It was fine. Then Peter put it in his ear. When he did, it was observed that he turned the aid down because his earmold no longer fit well and he objected to the feedback. He said, "The earmold doesn't fit well, but I thought it was perfect and I didn't want to bother my mother." (Most deaf kids use the word "perfect"). The audiologist phoned his mother, but she thought that because the earmold was only 6 months old it should fit and that Peter simply wasn't paying attention at home. The point is that the earmold should be checked as well as the hearing aid. A teacher or audiologist or parent should know what the children can hear with and without a hearing aid and then check each part to make sure that all parts are functioning. For example, some children don't put their ear-level aids in without twisting the tube. They don't set it in place. One must look at the child, see what he is doing, and then make an evaluation based on what the child can do.

PARENTS' NEED FOR INFORMATION

AUDIENCE MEMBER: Parents need to know that the earmolds have to fit well and they have to know basic facts about hearing aids. They should look at the aid to see if it's twisted. The parent dresses the child in the morning and should check the child before sending the child off to school.
DR. RUBIN: Maybe not the parent. Maybe an older sister. Sometimes the parent is working.
AUDIENCE MEMBER: Someone in the house should be responsible. The parents do not have enough information.
MRS. GRAMMATICO: I completely agree. We need some kind of on-going education for parents and for siblings. Deafness does not just affect one person; it affects the entire family. Our parent education is at night so we get both the parents and the siblings to come in. Also, the parents need to realize that teachers are not always going to be around. This is their responsibility. This was brought home to them at Peninsula Oral. I said, "We schedule 30 minutes of tutorial instruction per day, per child. If the hearing aid is not functioning, teachers have to take a part of your child's individual therapy time to do something about the hearing aid. If you bring it to me when your child enters school and tell me what's wrong with it, then teachers don't have to take any therapy time to replace it." This got through beautifully. Parents listened to hearing aids. Parents ought to know about frequency response, distortion, and how to measure it. When they pick up a hearing aid from a dealer, they ought to know how it is functioning. Parents are very capable of doing this. They are highly motivated to do it. They like being able to work out those graphs. I know. We do it year after year.

DR. RUBIN: Parents are given copies of our findings to bring in to a hearing aid dealer and say, "This is what is wrong with the hearing aid." In New York the parent explanation may be in English or Spanish. A good Spanish staff can explain, in very specific terms, how the aid works. Then they really communicate.

EXPECTATIONS FOR HEARING-IMPAIRED CHILDREN

DR. MADELL: We lose sight of how far hearing-impaired children can go, and, as Mrs. Grammatico said just a short while ago, "There are a lot of audiologists who have never had the opportunity to see successful hearing-impaired kids." That is unfortunate because it means that their goals for the kids are much lower than they ought to be. Of all the things that were discussed, I want to emphasize that kids don't function the same with *every* hearing aid. It is important to try different hearing aids for that reason, although the loaner aid programs present difficulty to lots of centers. From my point of view, it should not take 6 to 8 months once the hearing aid evaluation procedure has begun.

DR. ZANER: Even if it does not take 6 to 8 months, it's still inappropriate. For the same reasons that I mentioned earlier, it is inappropriate even if it takes 3 months. All the texts are suggesting that audiologists spend a month with each aid. My comments are in response, not necessarily to the very best of programs at the Lexington Hearing Center and at the New York League, but to what is going on in most places. Two months is a big chunk out of a preschool age child's language-acquisition time. It should not be wasted with undue manipulations because audiologists are not sure.

ACOUSTIC ENVIRONMENTS FOR HEARING-IMPAIRED CHILDREN

DR. ZANER: Dr. Rubin, you said something that I'm not sure I understood. If I did understand, I'm not sure I agree with it. You said that we need to look at a deaf child, as well as his hearing counterpart. Could you explain that more fully?

DR. RUBIN: My reason for making that remark is that, very frequently, we look at research that has been performed with the normal ear and then we say: "Oh, yes, if this happens with the normal ear we can infer that this will happen with the pathological ear." For example, in a classroom a normal hearing child can learn to discriminate when there is 60 dB of noise going on and can learn language without sound absorption material on the

136

walls and ceilings. He can learn to separate the signal from the ground in areas where the hearing-impaired child could not possibly function. One problem that an audiologist has is to choose amplification for children in specific educational settings. The hearing child can discriminate under circumstances which the hearing-impaired child cannot. The hearing-impaired child is going to be mainstreamed into a public school setting where there is a highly reverberant room and the child will not have an adequate input. Frequently, the only recommendation made is for preferential seating. That's a very minimal kind of accommodation for that hearing-impaired child. Many mainstreamed programs are developing in which the hearing-impaired child cannot learn. That is what I had in mind. My quotation, as I recall, was "that we need to look at him in his own environment." We need to look at the acoustic environment in which the child learns language and in which he listens. The closer the teacher or educator is to that child, the better signal he is going to get, and that doesn't happen in some schools.

DR. ZANER: I would certainly not disagree with that approach, but I would like to suggest a modification of it. There is a job that we, as professional educators, ought to think about for *every* child. To assume that a normal hearing child does well in a room that is not acoustically special, or visually special, is a fallacy. Schools are terrible places for children because schools put children in groups and assume that the children have to conform to the norm. That's not to say that they shouldn't be in school, but to say that a hearing-impaired child cannot be looked at as though he were normally hearing in terms of all those variables has to be modified to include saying that he has some *special* things that have to be looked at, in addition to all the other special things that all normally hearing children need.

MRS. GRAMMATICO: School is one of the most artificial situations that a child comes in contact with, next to the soundproof booth where he is tested. Certainly the signal that the hearing-impaired child gets has to be close. Our teachers work very closely with their children. They work on distance at a later time. They also use a strategy in the classroom whereby they ask the child, if he does not understand the auditory signal, to walk closer to the signal.

All children use their senses selectively as needed. The deaf child needs the opportunity to use his senses selectively as well as the hearing child. He also needs the opportunity to listen!

SUMMARY

Martha Rubin

The discussion on hearing aids for infants and children revealed divergent viewpoints on hearing aid evaluation among the participants and members of the audience. There were areas of agreement. Based on evidence that the hearing child was developing listening skills from the very first day of life, everyone agreed that early identification of hearing loss was critical. Dr. Rubin further emphasized the point that the hearing-impaired infant needed to be identified within the first 3 months of life and that there was an audiological and an educational responsibility to provide appropriate amplification soon thereafter.

PROGRAM AT LEXINGTON SCHOOL

Dr. Rubin described the program at the Lexington Hearing Center and co-jointly at the Lexington Infant Center which demonstrated the advantages of a total habilitative program for mother and child in a comprehensive educational setting.

It was noted that in New York State there has been a shift of responsibility for infants from a hospital setting to an educational setting because of the passage of the Baby Bill in 1973. The needs of the infant were shown to be very special because of the emerging mother-child relationship within the first 6 months of life. Audiologically, hearing-impaired infants required special modifications of ear-level aids, such as aids which were thinner, did not distort the helix, and had top microphones to cut down on acoustic feedback. Low frequency amplification for infants was questioned if hearing through 4,000 Hz could be shown. Impedance testing was suggested as an ongoing necessity during the first year of life because of the high incidence of middle ear pathology in infants.

PROGRAM AT NEW YORK LEAGUE FOR THE HARD OF HEARING

Dr. Madell described the ongoing procedures of hearing aid evaluations practiced at the New York League for the Hard of Hearing and cautioned against the fitting of binaural amplification for everyone. Trial periods of 2 to 3 months were suggested before hearing aid recommendations were made for children. The League's procedure was to keep a child on a loaner aid until the child showed some evidence of speech discrimination and could be tested using that evidence. A child with a profound loss, for example, might require more time than 3 months for a hearing aid evaluation. An interesting procedure developed at the league for children with only vibrotactile hearing was the use of a body aid with low frequency emphasis coupled to a bone-conduction vibrator strapped to the wrist.

PROGRAM AT MOUNT CARMEL GUILD

Dr. Zaner took issue with the entire concept of trial use of loaner hearing aids for preschool children. She pointed out that audiologists based their hearing aid procedures for children on an adult model. She preferred not to rely on noninstrumental criteria (the subjective preference of an aid based on teachers, parents, and clinicians reports). She stated that a long trial period and evaluation for the preschool child could be detrimental to the acquisition of language, and she advised that recommendations should be made in the form of a quick, firm decision by the audiologist, based on audiological assessment. She indicated that training institutions and the textbooks in use have perpetuated a mythical need for a trial loaner program for the preschool child, based on an adult model.

PROGRAM AT PENINSULA ORAL SCHOOL

Mrs. Grammatico described the development of listening skills based on cognitively rich educational content lessons. According to Mrs. Grammatico, children need to listen to speech and not to toy bells and drums and sound toys. They need to process information auditorily and re-organize the information that they bring from home. She suggested a sequential hierarchy of using songs, stories, sentences, phrases, words, and, last of all, elements for auditory training. She preferred to call auditory training "the development of listening skills." She noted that most professionals tend to use small words like "sad" with hearing-impaired children because small words are easily imitated. Such words carry very little acoustic information, compared with words that provide more acoustic information, such as "angry," "unhappy," or "frustrated." Deaf children need and can hear words like "frustrated." These are mood words which convey word color and voice color.

Mrs. Grammatico emphasized the use of the question, "What do you see?," which she said was the number one cognitive question to ask. She hoped that teachers would not accept one word answers, but would try to challenge a child's thinking. "Teachers really don't ask the right questions," she observed. "They ask questions to organize the information the way the teacher thinks the information should be organized as opposed to an educator who enables the learner (the child) to use the information that he or she has acquired from many different experiences." The development of listening skills as an ongoing process goes on *all* the time. She noted that, in her school, each child had three or four hearing aids in order to insure consistent amplification.

In the discussion period thereafter, there was a series of topics discussed such as auditory training units versus personal hearing aids, binaural amplification, and parent responsibilities. A consensus of opinion held that a prime need was for parent education. The responsibility for children's hearing aids should be shared not only by audiologists and educators—but also by parents because parents are the key to successful living for their children.

HEARING AID
EVALUATION
PROCEDURES

INTRODUCTION AND REVIEW OF HEARING AID EVALUATION PROCEDURES

Mark Ross

This presentation has all the characteristics of a projective test; each writer has expressed what the term "hearing aid evaluation procedure" meant to him. It would have been very ego gratifying if everybody agreed with everything, but our purposes have been better met since this was not the case and some contrary views were shared.

DEFINITION OF THE PROBLEM

The term "hearing aid evaluation procedures" sets up an orientation which we have to overcome. It was applicable 30 years ago when Carhart (1946) first described them. It is no tribute to him to find that most clinics are still essentially following the same procedures.

When these procedures were first described, little was known about the relationship between electroacoustic dimensions and speech intelligibility. The most effective way of selecting the "best" aid for a person—or at least ensuring that the patient didn't get the worst—was to administer a comparative hearing aid evaluation. The orientation this led to was that audiologists were looking for the best hearing aid for a person. Now it seems we should be defining the problem somewhat differently. Do we really care that brand X is better than brand Y? Or do we want to know, given a person's unique hearing loss characteristics, whether electro-acoustic pattern X is superior to pattern Y for this particular person? We should be focusing on those electroacoustic dimensions which have been shown to relate positively to intelligibility and then selecting, at least as a first step, those hearing aids which embody the desired characteristics. We are, it seems, in the paradoxical situation of recommending amplification, yet attending minimally, and denying the import of the characteristics of this amplification.

The important electroacoustic dimensions, and particularly their inter-action in specific instruments, have not been defined. Behavioral measures are still necessary as a validity check, but a great deal more is known than is practiced clinically, both in regard to electroacoustics and speech dis-crimination measures.

CURRENT PROBLEMS

Speech Discrimination Measures in Noise

The main reason that hearing aid evaluations are in disrepute in some quarters is the lack of reliability and sensitivity of the testing instrument: the speech discrimination measures. Yet how many audiologists employ a defensible degree of scientific rigor in approaching this problem? There is a lot of information, for example, which indicates that the simultaneous presence of a competing signal, from a spatially separated source, increases the sensitivity of our speech discrimination measures. However, in many instances, testing is still accomplished in a quiet situation only, and we wonder why our tests do not reflect known differences in electroacoustic dimensions. This is one example of clinical intertia, of being comfortable with a procedure and resisting any modification of it. All procedures, no matter what they are, have to be subjected to an ongoing critical appraisal to check for their current suitability.

Speech Discrimination Test Procedures: Write-Down Response

In this same respect, talk-back responses are accepted from patients, knowing even as we do that our own discrimination skills are being tested. The microphone in the test chamber may be 6 feet from the patient, his lips may not be visible, his speech may be terrible, and the competing signal may be at a disadvantageous signal to noise ratio. After doing all this, the complaint is that methodology is unreliable. Of course it is, under these conditions! For many patients, audiologists have to be flexible in their testing approach, yet, for the majority of them, write-down or cross-out responses are perfectly feasible.

Live Voice Testing

Finally, again in terms of testing, audiologists tend to prefer live voice testing, knowing even as we do that there are variations between talkers and even between the same talker on different days. There are any number of recorded lists available, but time and again I have observed audiologists' preference for live voice administration when there appeared to be no extenuating circumstances.

Test Presentation Levels

We often evaluate hearing aids at a 30- or 40-dB sensation level (SL), even for people with severe losses, and thereby saturate a large number of the aids evaluated. Consider the individual with unaided sound-field speech reception thresholds of 70 dB and aided thresholds of 20-dB HL (which is, incidently, a possible case of overfitting). When we administer discrimination tests at a 40-dB SL or 60-dB HL, we are actually presenting a stimulus of about 80-dB SPL. Coupled to the 50-dB gain, the sound pressure at the patient's ear is 130-dB SPL, if it hasn't saturated sooner. These lists should be presented at an average speech intensity level, about 65-dB SPL, or, at the most, at the patient's aided comfort level. Given the unrealistically high sound pressure levels used in comparative hearing aid evaluations, is it any wonder that results tend not to be too reliable?

Reference Levels

Another problem, which has been recognized by many people in the hearing aid industry for a number of years, is that audiologists have been victimized by two sets of reference levels. We have used audiograms, which use a zero hearing level as a reference, to select hearing aids, the electro-acoustics of which are defined in terms of another reference level, sound pressure level re 0.0002 dynes/cm^2. Since the acoustics of speech are also usually described in sound pressure level terms, we have been in the position of mixing pears and peaches and wondering why the product isn't applesauce. My suggestion is that we express all behavioral and electro-acoustic measures and dimensions in a sound pressure level scale. Some problems will still remain, particularly in respect to the coupler effect, but not as many. We define the characteristics of the aid in terms of a 2-cc coupler and then deliver the signal into an ear canal which may or may not act like the coupler at all. Here, it is not a question of which coupler is best, the new ones being recommended or the ones incorporated in the KEMAR artificial head, but just the fact that any coupler is at best an approximation of real ear characteristics. Ultimately, we have to measure what is going on in the real ear and then relate these measures to intelligibility scores.

SOME KNOWN—BUT LITTLE USED—INFORMATION

First, we have been overfitting patients for years. "Use" gain turns out to be about half of the patient's hearing threshold level. Two recent articles, one in the "British Journal of Audiology" (1973), and one in "Scandanavian Audiology" (1975), point this out. Geary McCandless has done the most extensive work in this area and will report on this factor in more detail in his paper.

Upward Spread of Masking

Second, a high-pass signal will increase intelligibility for most patients. This is supported by the work of Danaher, Osberger, and Pickett (1973), who demonstrated an upward spread of masking and a perceptual effect of low frequencies upon the perception of higher frequency, second formant transitions. Thomas and Sparks (1975) showed that hearing-impaired listeners increased their intelligibility scores when exposed to high-pass, peak-clipping processing of the speech signal. The relatively large number of studies showing that open-mold or no-mold fittings for hearing-impaired subjects improve their intelligibility scores, particularly under noise conditions, also supports this assertion. It will be recalled that the acoustical effect of an open-mold fitting is essentially that of a high-pass filter. And, finally, studies at the Central Institute for the Deaf (Pascoe, Niemoeller, and Miller, 1973) demonstrated that an increase in intelligibility resulted when the high frequency acoustical resonances of the external auditory meatus were provided to the patient by an amplifier unit.

High Frequency Amplification

Third, the extension of the high frequency range of hearing aids, much past the usual 3,000 Hz, can prove beneficial to many hearing-impaired people. Until recently, the upper range of wearable hearing aids precluded the perception of all or some of many high frequency phonemes. Adults were, thus, deprived of potentially valuable information, although perhaps redundant for them, while children, with no previous knowledge of the language to call on, were compelled to try to develop an auditory-based language system, with many of the potentially audible elements filtered out by the hearing aid. That the higher frequencies can assist in speech discrimination was demonstrated by Geary McCandless and by Pascoe, Niemoeller, and Miller (1973).

Threshold of Discomfort

Finally, probably the most important, but little used, information relates to control of the maximum output of hearing aids. Audiologists should be measuring the threshold of *beginning* discomfort, frequency by frequency, and limit the output of our hearing aids accordingly.

SUMMARY

My basic thesis in this brief discussion is that electroacoustic characteristics are important, that they do relate to intelligibility, and that more energy should be devoted to selecting those electroacoustic dimensions which can most effectively process a speech signal, and package them, as best we can, to the measured aberrations of a particular individual's hearing problem. Ed Villchur, who has done the most sophisticated work in signal processing, will present his work later in this book. Until work like his, however, becomes clinically practicable and available, audiologists are still faced with an essentially trial and error procedure in clinics. This is not to say that every hearing aid evaluation has to be a "tabula rasa," that we have to begin each evaluation completely from scratch. There is much information, as has been demonstrated, but we do have to support our judgments with behavioral measures. Again, behavioral measures have to be scientifically defensible and provide us with some validity assurances when the evaluation is completed.

LITERATURE CITED

Brooks, D. 1973. Gain requirements of hearing aid users. Scand. Audiol. 2: 199–204.

Carhart, R. 1946. Tests for selection of hearing aids. Laryngoscope 56: 780–794.

Danaher, E. M., M. J. Osberger, and J. M. Pickett. 1973. Discrimination of formant frequency transitions in synthetic vowels. J. Speech & Hearing Res. 16: 439–451.

Martin, M. C. 1973. Hearing aid gain requirements in sensori-neural hearing loss. Brit. J. Audiol. 7: 21–34.

Pascoe, D. P., A. F. Niemoeller, and J. D. Miller. 1973. Hearing aid design and evaluation for a presbycusic patient. Presented at the 86th meeting of the Acoustical Society of America.

Ross, M. 1975. Hearing aid selection for the preverbal hearing-impaired child. *In* M. Pollack (ed.), Amplification for the Hearing Impaired. Grune & Stratton, Inc., New York.

Thomas, I. W., and D. W. Sparks. 1975. Discrimination of filtered/clipped speech by hearing-impaired subjects. J. Acoust. Soc. Amer. 49: 1881–1887.

PRESCRIPTIVE FITTING OF WEARABLE MASTER HEARING AIDS: A PROGRESS REPORT

H. Levitt, R. E. C. White, and S. B. Resnick

PURPOSE

The purpose of this project is to develop a practical protocol for the prescriptive fitting of a wearable master hearing aid (WMHA). The WMHAs used in this study were developed by Bolt, Beraneck, and Newman under contract for the National Institute of Neurological and Communicative Diseases and Stroke. The instrument is pocket-sized (outer dimensions are 5.5 X 3.25 X 1 inches), weighs 6 ounces, and can be worn conveniently in a vestpocket or similar location with leads running to the ears for connection to conventional hearing aid receivers and microphones. There are two separate channels for binaural amplification with a variety of plug-in units for modifying the characteristics of the hearing aid. By suitable choice of plug-in units, it is possible to change the frequency response, compression and/or clipping characteristics, gain, maximum power output, and other relevant variables of the hearing aid over a wide range of parameter values.

PROGRESS TO DATE

At the time of writing, the project for developing a practical protocol for prescriptive fitting of the WMHA had been active for 9 months, the project having begun July 1, 1974. The following was accomplished during this period:

1. The seven WMHAs to be used in the project were checked and calibrated.
2. A pool of potential subjects was assembled from the records of participating clinics.
3. A comprehensive set of test materials was prepared, including an appropriate phoneme discrimination test.
4. An experimental test protocol was established.
5. Two pilot subjects were run through the basic test battery.

A summary of the work accomplished in each of the above areas follows.

Calibration of Units

Calibration procedures were formalized which, in general, corresponded with the recommendations of ANSI Standard S3.3 (1960). The basic calibration information obtained on each aid included: (1) frequency gain characteristics for all linear modules, (2) checks on the linearity of the gain control, (3) pressure and free-field calibration of microphones, including a check of directional characteristics, and, (4) 2-cc coupler calibration of transducers.

In order to allow convenient spot checks of the units, a test fixture has been built which allows for the direct connection of electrical signals to the input of the WMHA. This arrangement provides for more convenient testing of all aspects of the WMHA, except for that of the microphone itself. It has the important advantage that testing is much more rapid and reliable calibration checks of the WMHA can be obtained by relatively inexperienced persons, since it removes the need for careful control of an acoustic environment. Each test fixture consists of a shielded box containing a field effect transister which simulates the preamplifier associated with each microphone, together with an input connector to fit the WMHA.

Use of the KEMAR Manikin

Calibration of the insert receiver using the KEMAR manikin reveals considerable differences between frequency response curves with a standard 2-cc coupler and those made with the same insert receiver worn by the manikin. The reasons for this are not yet clear; however, there is some evidence that one effect of an earmold is to cause the external ear canal to resonate at a frequency on the order of 1 to 2 kilohertz. The location of this resonance may depend critically on the manner of insertion of the mold and might vary as the mold is removed and replaced in day-to-day use. This potential variability suggests that attempts to cancel this resonance by the design of special plug-in modules with individually tailored frequency response may be difficult, and the perfect cancellation is unlikely. Nevertheless, initial inquiries have been made regarding the possible use of such special modules.

It has been suggested that it may be possible to modify an earphone by the addition of an acoustical network in such a way that the resultant acoustical impedance is matched to the characteristic impedance of the ear canal (Wallace, 1975). If such impedance matching can be made reasonably stable, then the problem of resonant behavior mentioned above would disappear.

A second approach being taken is an ancillary project designed to investigate the perceptual importance of such resonances. This study would attempt to estimate the extent to which such resonances have a measurable effect on speech intelligibility. The results would indicate the acceptable magnitude of impedance mismatch between earphone and ear.

Selection of Subjects

All patient records at the five clinics within the city university system have been examined. In addition, the New York League for the Hard of Hearing has kindly offered to help provide subjects for this study, and we have been permitted to review their patient records. The records of all potential subjects have been collated and cross-referenced with respect to the variables of interest in this project. The pool of potential subjects now numbers over 300 hearing-impaired individuals, representing a broad spectrum of hearing loss and past experience with amplification. Prospective subjects for the first test group (i.e., individuals with moderate bilateral symmetrical hearing loss) have been contacted and are participating in the study.

Preparation of Test Material

The test material was chosen to cover a wide range of speech reception tasks, including phoneme discrimination, monosyllabic word discrimination, sentence reception, and understanding of continuous discourse. Where possible, tests that were readily available have been used (MRHT, CHABA sentences, ratings of intelligibility of connected discourse). For the important case of phoneme discrimination, a suitable test was not available and a special monosyllabic nonsense syllable test was developed. The test is described in the Appendix. The advantage of this test is that it is a balanced closed-response-set test, in which the choice of foils is based on minimal assumptions regarding what the subject might perceive. The only assumption needed to reduce the set of foils to a manageable size is that voiced/voiceless confusions are relatively infrequent and may be omitted from the set of foils without biasing the results unduly. This assumption is based on a review of the published literature which shows this error to be one of the least frequent discrimination errors for hearing-impaired listeners.

Recordings were made of all tests by both a male speaker and a female speaker. The speakers were selected by a trained phonetician (Dr. William Stewart) with considerable experience in dialectology. The criteria for selection included dialect, voice quality, and control.

All master recordings have been equalized for level, and submasters have been prepared which are used to generate test tapes as needed. The submasters include different randomizations of the test material, as well as various distortions of the speech material, such as reverberation and the addition of background noise. The noise tape prepared for use in this study consists of segments selected from a tape recording made in a crowded cafeteria. The segments selected consist primarily of the simultaneous conversations of a number of male and female speakers and are relatively constant in level. The tape has been edited only to remove passages of clearly intelligible speech and extreme transient sounds. Conditions of reverberation are simulated by rerecording the standard test tapes via a loudspeaker and a microphone placed in an uncarpeted, modestly furnished room.

Experimental Test Protocol: Baseline Audiometric Data

An experimental test protocol consisting of five stages has been established. Stage I is devoted to the acquisition of baseline audiometric data. Stage II involves the administration of a battery of 36 diagnostic tests; 32 of these tests form a basic Latin Square design, the remaining four tests make up a 2 X 2 factorial design consisting of permutations of the best and second best estimates, respectively, of the optimum amplitude and frequency-response characteristics, as obtained from the Latin Square analysis. The best of these estimates is then used as the initial hearing aid setting for the convergence phase.

EXPERIMENTAL DESIGN

The experimental design used in Stage II is summarized in Table 1 and Figure 1. Table 1 shows a listing of the three factors making up the Latin Square design. Factor A consists of various combinations of amplitude characteristics. Note that settings A_1 to A_4 consist of compression condi-

Table 1. Dimensions of Latin-Square design

Factor A: amplitude dimension (8 levels)

Level	Compressor	Compressor type	Decay time	Clipping type	MPO
A_1	Present	Full	20 msec	Hard	115
A_2	Present	Full	100 msec	Hard	115
A_3	Present	Knee	20 msec	Hard	115
A_4	Present	Knee	100 msec	Hard	115
A_5	Absent			Hard	110
A_6	Absent			Hard	120
A_7	Absent			Soft	110
A_8	Absent			Soft	120

(Note: attack time fixed at 10 msec)

Factor B: frequency dimension (4 levels)

B_1	0 dB Slope
B_2	+6 dB Slope
B_3	−6 dB Slope
B_4	0 dB Slope—band limited 500–3,000 Hz

Factor C: listening mode

C_1	Quiet
C_2	Noise[a]
C_3	Reverberation
C_4	Noise (with speaker of opposite sex)

[a]For the testing conditions employing noise in this study, the noise level is adjusted so that the level of peaks within the noise is about 10 dB below that of speech.

tions and that A_5 to A_8 consist of clipping conditions. Factor B consists of various frequency-response settings and Factor C consists of four major conditions which affect listening performance but which are not controlled directly by settings of the WMHA. Three of the four conditions covered by Factor C cover speech reception for a given speaker in quiet, noise, and reverberation, respectively. The fourth condition is a repetition of the noise condition with a speaker of the opposite sex. Half of the subjects will have a female speaker for conditions C_1 to C_3, the other half of the subjects will have a male speaker for these three conditions. Figure 1 shows the basic experimental design. Two symmetrical Latin Squares are used, one covering the compression conditions A_1 to A_4, the other covering the clipping conditions A_5 to A_8. Discrimination scores on the

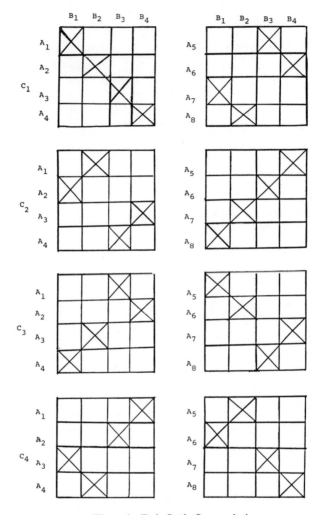

Figure 1. Twin Latin-Square design.

Nonsense Syllable Test and ratings of connected discourse are obtained for each cell in the design.

Performance Comparisons

Stage III provides a comparison of performance in different types of test. This stage has been included so that the various tests used in the study may be compared with each other as well as with other tests used in studies of this type, such as Pascoe's High Frequency Word Test and the

MRHT. The comparative measurements are obtained in six selected cells spanning the range from two of the best conditions to two intermediate conditions to two of the worst conditions. Stage III is designed to provide information on the protocol itself and will not be included in the final protocol to be used by clinics in fitting hearing aids.

Convergence Phase

Stage IV covers the convergence phase. The subject is fitted with the WMHA set to the best estimate of the optimum hearing aid settings, as obtained from Stage II. The aid is then worn for a week, after which the subject returns for a reassessment of the aid's performance, followed by small, systematic variations on each hearing aid parameter to determine if an optimum has been reached. If an optimum has not been reached, a new estimate for the optimum setting is obtained, using a standard hill-climbing optimization procedure.

RESULTS OF EXPERIMENTAL PROCEDURE

The fifth and final stage is designed to estimate the improvement in performance attributable to the adjustment procedure and also to assess any learning effects. A comparison of the subject's performance with his own aid and the final estimate of the best setting of the WMHA is used to indicate the relative success of the experimental procedure. The comparison is made both in terms of other standard tests (W-22 discrimination test and MRHT). In addition, aided noise band thresholds are obtained to provide some insight as to the signals actually being received by the listener for the different aids.

Pilot Tests

Two subjects participated in a pilot study to test the feasibility of the experimental protocol. One of the subjects withdrew temporarily because of illness requiring hospitalization and will return as soon as she recovers. She is currently close to completion of Stage II of the experimental protocol. The second subject had reached convergence in one mode of operation of the aid (compression) and was to be tested for convergence in a second mode of operation (clipping) at the time of writing. Since the early part of the protocol was completed satisfactorily, with no major problems, it was decided to begin full-scale testing. Final convergence for the pilot subjects should be reached well before the first group of subjects completes Stage II of the protocol, and any changes for the latter part of the protocol, if so indicated by the pilot study, can be accomplished well in advance of the regular subjects reaching the latter stages of the protocol.

Acoustic feedback was encountered with the WMHA under certain conditions during the convergence stage. To avoid delaying the study, an immediate solution to the feedback problem was obtained by mounting the microphone as for a conventional body aid. The convergence phase was then restarted with the new microphone position. A more satisfactory solution to the problem of acoustic feedback is to improve the shielding of the acoustic signals, and this is currently being tried out.

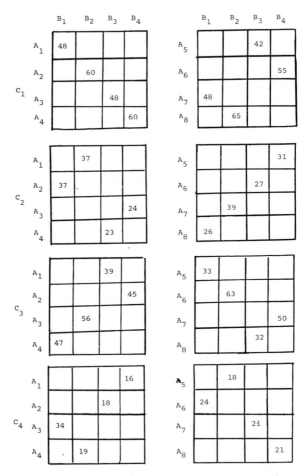

Figure 2. Subject 1. Amplitude, A: A_1, 35%; A_2, 40%; A_3, 40.5%; A_4, 373.%; A_5, 31%; A_6, 42.3%; A_7, 39.5%; A_8, 36%; A_{1-4}, 38.2%; A_{5-8}, 37.2%. Frequency, B: B_1, 37.2%; B_2, 44.7%; B_3, 31.3%; B_4, 37.8%. Listening mode, C: C_1, 53.5%; C_2, 30.6%; C_3, 45.7%; C_4, 21.4%. Overall $\bar{X}$, 37.7%.

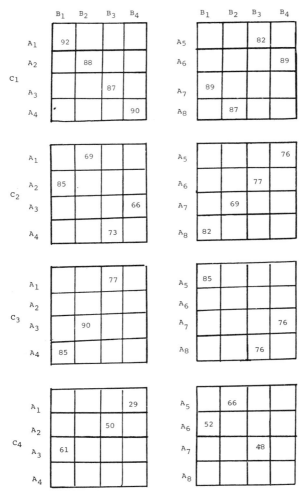

Figure 3. Subject 2. Amplitude, A: A_1, 78%; A_2, 75%; A_3, 76%; A_4, 83%; A_5, 77%; A_6, 73%; A_7, 70%; A_8, 82%. $A_{1\rightarrow4}$, 74.5%; $A_{5\rightarrow8}$, 75.3%. Frequency, B: B_1, 77%; B_2, 78%; B_3, 72%; B_4, 71%. Listening mode, C: C_1, 89%; C_2, 74%; C_3, 82%; C_4, 51%. Overall $\overline{X}$, 74.9%.

The data for the two pilot subjects obtained in Stage II of the protocol, the major data collection stage, are shown in Figures 2 and 3. These data show a fairly clear picture of which variables are important for each subject. Furthermore, although changes in the WMHA settings affected the subjects in different ways, there is evidence of a consistent pattern. In terms of frequency response, subject 1 performed best at a slope of +6 dB octave (setting B_2 as defined in Table 1), while subject 2 performed best, for the most part, at a flat frequency response, (i.e., 0 dB/octave, setting B_1). The negative slope of −6 dB/octave (setting B_3) was uniformly bad for both subjects.

The effects of changes in the amplitude dimension are less clear. While one setting can be chosen which yields the highest discrimination score, there are other settings involving completely different modes of operation of the aid (e.g., clipping versus compression) which yield similar discrimination scores. Subject 1 is in the convergence phase, and data currently being gathered suggest that there may be at least two major peaks in the discrimination surface. One peak appears to occur under conditions of compression, the other peak appears to occur in clipping mode. If this result is obtained consistently with other subjects, then the convergence strategy may need to be modified to allow for efficient selection of the higher of the two possible peaks.

CURRENT STATUS: FULL-SCALE TESTING

Full-scale testing with the complete experimental test protocol is under way on the first group of subjects. The experimental protocol in its present form provides extensive coverage of the variables that might be relevant to the development of a practical protocol for prescriptive fitting of wearable master hearing aids. It is anticipated that, as testing progresses, it will become apparent which aspects of the protocol provide the most information with respect to converging on the optimum set of parameter values for the hearing aid. It is planned to trim the experimental protocol to a manageable size for clinical use once sufficient data have been gathered to justify omitting those items which have been found consistently to yield the least information.

LITERATURE CITED

Wallace, R. W., Sr. 1975. New kind of headphone receivers. Paper (#HH1) presented at the 89th meeting of the Acoustical Society of America, April, Bell Laboratories, Murray Hill, N. J.

APPENDIX

Nonsense Syllable Test

The Nonsense Syllable Test is a closed response test consisting of CV, VC, and CVC syllables, organized into 12 modules. All but one of the modules are designed to provide information on the discriminability of consonants.

The subjects' responses to syllables within a given module are limited to other syllables within the same module. The construction of the modules was based on information regarding the frequency of occurrence of phoneme identification errors by normal-hearing and hearing-impaired individuals. The subject, therefore, has the opportunity to make errors of manner and place in phoneme identification within each module, but errors of voicing are not possible.

Seven modules of the test are being administered under all experimental conditions. Modules 1, 2, and 3 are designed to provide information on the discriminability of final unvoiced phonemes in three vowel contexts; /i/, /a/, and /u/. Module 4 permits assessment of the discriminability of final voiced phonemes in the /a/ context. The discriminability of initial phonemes is evaluated in module 5; modules 6 and 7 allow evaluation of discriminability of initial voiced phonemes.

The optional modules 1, 2, 3, and 4 are designed to provide information on the effect of: (1) discrimination of initial unvoiced phonemes as affected by vowel context; and (2) discrimination of final voiced phonemes as affected by vowel context. Optional module 5 was incorporated in the test to permit evaluation of the effects of amplification on vowel identification. It is anticipated that these effects will be minimal.

Nonsense Syllable Test

1	2	3	4	5	6	7
af	uθ	iʃ	að	fa	la	na
aʃ	up	if	ab	ta	ba	va
at	us	it	am	pa	da	ma
ak	uk	ik	az	ha	ga	za
as	ut	is	ag	θa	ra	ga
ap	uf	iθ	an	tʃa	ja	ba
aθ	uʃ	ip	av	sa	dʒa	ða
				ʃa	wa	da
				ka		

Optional Modules

1	2	3	4	5
ʃu	tʃi	ið	uz	kip
fu	ʃi	ib	ub	kap
su	pi	iv	uð	kup
ku	si	iz	uv	kæp
tʃu	hi	id	um	pet
θu	θi	ig	un	pɪt
hu	fi	in	un	pit
tu	ti	iŋ	ud	pæt
pu	ki	im	ug	

SIGNAL PROCESSING FOR HEARING AIDS

Edgar Villchur

Persons suffering from sensorineural deafness commonly find it difficult to understand speech even after it is amplified, and what understanding they do have is easily destroyed by acoustical interference. The analogy developed in this paper suggests that recruitment, which exaggerates the loudness differences that the deaf subject perceives among the acoustical elements of speech, is a sufficient cause for both of these difficulties.

SIGNAL PROCESSING TO SIMULATE RECRUITMENT

The *dashed lines* in Figure 1 outline the approximate sound pressure levels of conversational speech, measured in ½-octave bands by Dunn and White (1940). The speech band is plotted against the dynamic range of normal hearing for speech, between threshold and the ISO 74-phon equal-loudness contour.

The *upper left portion* of Figure 2 shows the deaf-subject equivalent of the normal hearing span that we saw in Figure 1. The *solid lines* mark the average of the thresholds, and equal-loudness contours related to preferred speech levels, of six deaf subjects. These data were measured in a previous experiment (Villchur, 1973). The reduced dynamic range of the deaf subjects' hearing reflects their recruitment. Plotted against this band of residual hearing is the amplified speech band.

The processed speech in the graph *on the right* in Figure 2 is a projection of the amplified speech from the abnormal to the normal hearing span, keeping the proportionate relationships between speech levels and hearing spans the same. Each acoustical element of speech, at

161

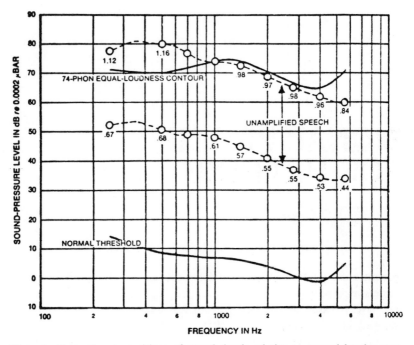

Figure 1. Proportionate positions of speech levels relative to normal hearing span. (Villchur, 1973.)

each frequency/amplitude coordinate of the amplified speech band at the left, is projected to the same relative level in the normal span of hearing as this element has in the deaf-subject span. Thus, if the hearing-span analogy is valid, the loudness relationships perceived by a normal listener in the processed speech will be the same as the loudness relationships perceived by the deaf subjects in the amplified but unprocessed speech. Two check points of the analogy may be noted—for both normals and deaf subjects, the extreme speech levels drop below threshold at the same frequencies, 1.2 kilohertz for the lowest-level speech elements and 3.1 kilohertz for the highest-level speech elements. To put it another way, those elements of speech that are inaudible to the deaf subjects will also be inaudible to the normal listener. A detailed discussion of this analogy has been published (Villchur, 1974).

ELECTRONIC SIMULATOR

This processing of speech to simulate the loudness relationships heard by the deaf subjects can be realized in practice by subjecting the speech signal to fast-acting, frequency-dependent volume expansion, followed by treble attenuation. A three-channel version of the circuit of Figure 3 was used.

The *solid dots at the right* in Figure 2 indicate the accuracy of processing that was achieved for discrete signals. The validity of the processing for complex signals has been supported by an experiment with

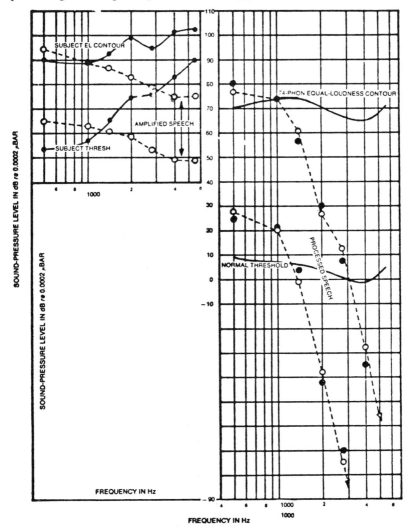

Figure 2. Projection of the amplified speech band from the deaf-subject span of hearing to the normal span, keeping the same proportionate relationship between speech levels and corresponding hearing spans. *Solid dots* show actual processing. (Villchur, 1974.)

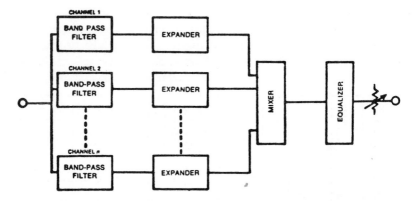

Figure 3. Idealized signal processor to simulate for normal listeners the abnormal loudness relationships perceived by a deaf subject with recruitment. The processor is an electrical analog of recruitment. The electrical response of the model represents the deaf subject's loudness response relative to normal response. (Villchur, 1974.)

four subjects, each with unilateral deafness and recruitment, who compared the simulation with the real thing, that is, they compared individually processed speech in the normal ear with unprocessed speech amplified to the same loudness in the impaired ear. The subjects reported the two signals to be similar or very similar in quality, but dissimilar when processing was removed from the normal-ear signal.

Hearing Aid Compensation

The processed speech in Figure 2 can be processed again to simulate the hearing aid compensation that was used in an earlier experiment with these deaf subjects—two-band, frequency-dependent amplitude compression followed by treble boost.

The *solid dots* and *heavy dashes on the right* in Figure 4 are a plot of the expanded/equalized speech corrected only by the high frequency-boost component of the compensation. As may be seen, the low-amplitude speech elements are not amplified to useful levels.

In Figure 5, the *solid dots* and *heavy dashes* mark the speech band reprocessed by compression only. The low-amplitude elements of speech are brought into the correct loudness relationship with high amplitude elements of the same frequency, but severe high frequency attenuation remains.

Compression/Equalization

For subjects with recruitment, compression without postcompression equalization may restore enough acoustical information for listening to speech under ideal conditions, but not enough for the listener to tolerate destructive influences like interference or reverberation. The limited number of recognition cues that have been made available to the deaf subjects do not include a reserve against further losses.

In Figure 6, the *solid dots* and *heavy dashes* show the speech band

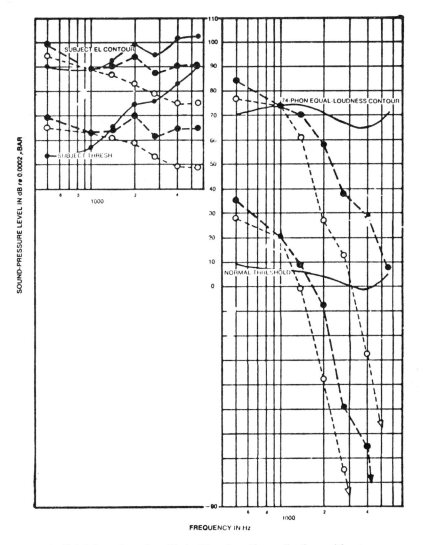

Figure 4. *Solid dots* show the effect of hearing-aid equalizations without compression. (Villchur, 1974.)

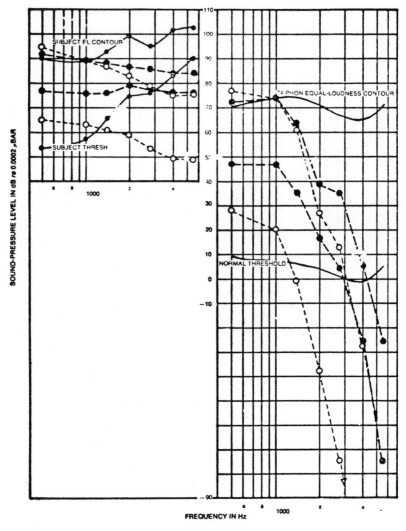

Figure 5. *Solid dots* show the effect of compression without equalization. (Villchur, 1974.)

reprocessed by both compression and post-compression equalization to an imperfect copy of the normal speech band in Figure 1. This hearing aid processing will restore near-normal intensity relationships to the transposed speech shown *at the right* in Figure 2, which means that, if the recruitment analogy is valid, the circuit will process normal, amplified speech to have near-normal loudness relationships for the deaf subject represented at the *upper left* of Figure 2. The separate elements of speech are amplified to the appropriate relative levels within his hearing span.

Compression and Post-compression Frequency Equalization

The analogy suggests that the use of both compression and post-compression frequency equalization in a hearing aid designed for subjects with

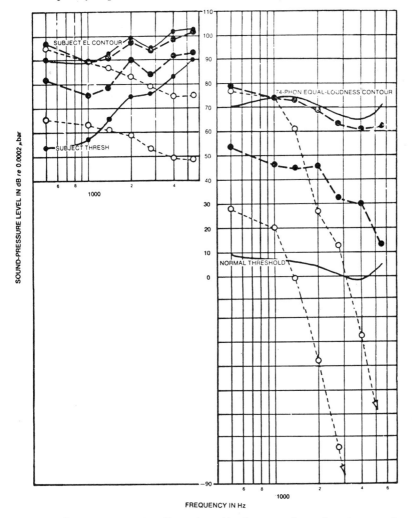

Figure 6. *Solid dots* show the effect of combined compression and postcompression equalization. (Villchur, 1974.)

recruitment is likely to have considerably greater benefit than the arithmetic sum of the separate, limited benefits of each process, particularly in the presence of interference. Either process by itself may have the unrewarding effect of lifting critical elements of speech from well below the subject's threshold to just below that threshold.

Hypotheses, rather than conclusions, are properly derived from the analogy, and these hypotheses must be tested in the real world of deaf subjects. The earlier experiment with the six deaf subjects whose recruitment was simulated does lend support to these hypotheses.

Figure 7 is from that earlier report. Here compression plus treble boost projects the speech band from the normal to the abnormal hearing span of one of the subjects—the reverse of the recruitment-simulation process. The proportionate relationships between speech levels and hearing spans are again kept the same, this time so that the deaf subjects can perceive the same loudness relationships among the acoustical elements of speech as are perceived by normal listeners. Speech recognition for all six subjects was improved significantly by this type of processing, and when a background of competing speech was added to the intelligibility tests—the interference being equally subject to the processing—the benefit of the processing to speech intelligibility was usually increased.

Combined Distortions

Martin, Murphy, and Meyer (1956) reported that, when speech was subjected to high frequency attenuation similar to that in the compressed-only speech of Figure 5, not much of the intelligibility was lost for normal listeners in a quiet environment. However, when the same treble attenuation was combined with other distortions, such as multiple echoes and/or noise, each relatively innocuous by itself, intelligibility was reduced significantly. The hearing aid user listens in an environment that includes reverberation, noise, and competing speech, and his perceptive aberrations combine with external distortions.

SUMMARY

Two major problems that must be considered by the designer of hearing aids for the perceptively deaf are poor subject recognition of amplified, clear speech and the abnormal vulnerability of this reduced recognition to acoustical interference. Signal processing that relieves the first problem may simultaneously relieve the second, by restoring redundant speech recognition cues to the subject's preception. The experiment with actual deaf subjects referred to earlier lends support to such a conclusion.

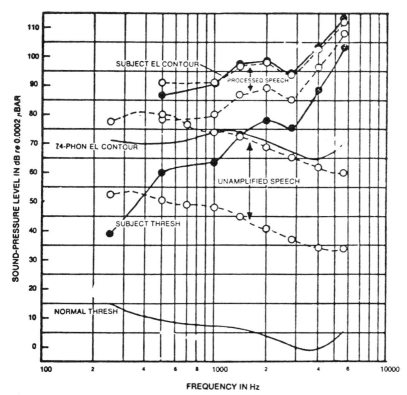

Figure 7. Calculated compression/equalization processing for a deaf subject with recruitment. The reference level of the deaf subject equal-loudness contour is related to that of the 74-phon contour by way of the deaf subject's preferred listening level for speech. (Villchur, 1974.)

LITERATURE CITED

Dunn, H. W., and S. D. White. 1940. Statistical measurements on conversational speech. J. Acoust. Soc. Amer. 11: 278–288.

Martin, D. W., R. L. Murphy, and A. Meyer. 1956. Articulation reduction by combined distortions of speech waves. J. Acoust. Soc. Amer. 28: 597–601.

Villchur, E. 1973. Signal processing to improve speech intelligibility in perceptive deafness. J. Acoust. Soc. Amer. 53: 1646–1657.

Villchur, E. 1974. Simulation of the effect of recruitment on loudness relationships in speech. J. Acoust. Soc. Amer. 56: 1601–1611.

SPECIAL CONSIDERATIONS IN EVALUATING CHILDREN AND THE AGING FOR HEARING AIDS

Geary A. McCandless

It is not the intent of this paper to discuss the relative value of the numerous clinical techniques used in selection of hearing aids. Rather, the objective is to examine and challenge some of the basic assumptions and practices currently in vogue and to suggest basic tests which can be used to assess and predict aided function.

This paper is further intended to illustrate the necessity of considering each hearing loss individually. That is, to show that audiometrically similar hearing loss may represent vastly different pathologies, therefore, they will have differing functional residual. This paper will deal with suggested measurements to specify function and special considerations in hearing aid fitting as they relate to the geriatric patient and to children.

FAULTY ASSUMPTIONS IN HEARING AID FITTING

The clinician normally makes basic assumptions regarding the characteristics of the hearing loss in the process of coupling a hearing aid to the ear. If these basic assumptions are correct, the patient derives considerable

benefit. If the basic assumptions are erroneous, little benefit comes from
the use of a hearing aid. Since complaints from patients with hearing aids
are extremely common, one must assume either that the pathological ear
simply is not amenable to the introduction of a hearing aid or that some of
the basic assumptions regarding the character of the ear with pathology are
faulty.

Threshold of Discomfort

An example of this is the common concept that if a hearing aid is
introduced to an ear, the loud and somewhat annoying sounds first
experienced by the patient will subside as the ear gets "toughened up."
There is little or no substantive evidence to suggest that the ear will
tolerate louder sounds over time. The bulk of evidence suggests the
contrary, that is, the hearing aid user will set the gain at a lower level after
a period of use than during the initial evaluation. Such faulty assumptions
regarding the nature of the pathological ear have persisted for many years
and account for many of the failures to achieve reasonable satisfaction for
many hearing aid users.

BASIC ASSUMPTIONS RELATED TO THE IMPAIRED EAR

Gain Requirements

With any hearing impairment, there is a loss of sensitivity or acuity to soft
sounds which can be functionally restored at least in part by amplification.
While this observation appears obvious, the assumption that the soft
sounds can be totally reintroduced by increasing the gain by way of a
hearing aid may not be correct. For example, if a patient has an unaided
speech threshold of 50-dB HL, a typical aided threshold might be 20 dB.
The functional gain at a comfortable setting with the aid would be 30 dB.
The most common error by clinicians lies in the assumption that, if
hearing loss is 50 dB, for example, an attempt should be made to normalize
the hearing loss by introducing as near a 50-dB gains as possible, thus reducing functional acuity to zero. This goal cannot be realistically achieved
with present instrumentation because of the reduced dynamic range.

Distortion within the Auditory System

With most hearing impairment, considerable distortion is produced by the
pathological changes within the auditory system. The type and amount of
distortion depend on the pathology and severity of hearing loss. The
majority of candidates for hearing aids have cochlear type pathology.
Distortion within the cochlea is best characterized by the presence of

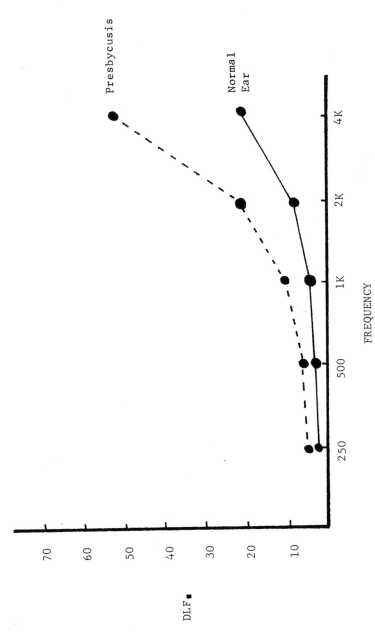

Figure 1. Difference limen for frequency (*DLF*) in a group of subjects with presbycusis and a group of normal subjects. The resolving power for frequency is seen to be significantly poorer in the presbycusic group.

recruitment, the few exceptions being of congenital hearing loss caused by hereditary or other factors. Other types of distortion may be equally severe, however. For example, diplacusis or other types of frequency distortion may occur; that is, the subject may lose the ability to differentiate between small changes in frequency as shown in Figure 1. There is also reason to believe there may be harmonic or other distortions present in the ear with pathology.

A hearing aid can compensate somewhat for the loss of sensitivity by making sounds louder. However, a hearing aid cannot restore frequency distortion inherent in the pathological ear. Indeed, the hearing aid may produce compounding effects when coupled to the pathological ear.

Functional Tolerance Thresholds

In most subjects, especially those with cochlear pathology, the upper usable tolerance limits (functional tolerance thresholds) are about the same as in the normal ear.

Results of Mismeasurement of Tolerance Threshold

Although the hearing loss may be severe, there may be little or no change in the point of beginning discomfort as compared with normal. The threshold of loudness discomfort should be carefully examined, since recent studies indicate that clinicians have grossly overestimated the tolerance levels of the pathological ear because of faulty techniques of measuring tolerance. As a consequence, excessive gain and maximum power output are recommended.

Whereas a majority of hearing aids on the market today are capable of producing sound pressures in excess of 125 dB, individuals with hearing losses even up to 75 and 80 dB will rarely tolerate sound pressures of 120 dB over a period of time. The chronic complaint of annoyance to loud sounds is understandable if indeed excessive sound pressure is being delivered to the ear. The reason for many of these complaints is that clinicians assume that the ear is able to tolerate sound pressures in excess of 120 dB and, in some cases, as high as 140 dB. Figure 2 illustrates the average tolerance level for speech as a function of hearing loss. It can be seen that the upper comfort limits change relatively little with hearing loss.

Hearing Aid Rejection Caused by Excessive MPO

About 50% of hearing aid users complain of some discomfort caused by excessive sound pressure to the ear, and 20 to 35% of hearing aid wearers restrict the use of their aids to part-time or reject them completely because of loudness discomfort. The most important single factor in hearing aid

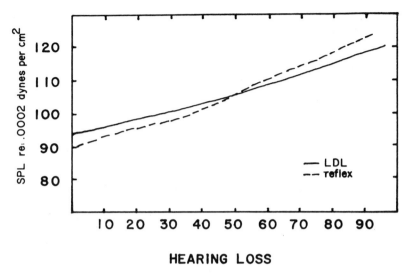

HEARING LOSS

Figure 2. The average thresholds of loudness discomfort for speech as a function of hearing loss. Acoustic reflex thresholds are also shown.

rejections is probably related to excessive power output of the aid. Care should be taken to determine the loudness discomfort threshold (not the threshold of pain) and limit the output accordingly.

DETERMINATION OF NEED FOR A HEARING AID

While the pure tone audiogram has for years been used as a basic criteria for determining the need for hearing aids, because of the variances of configuration and severity, this technique can be misleading. The following procedure is suggested regardless of the severity of loss and is a simple technique which can be used to answer the first and most important basic question, "Can the patient profit from amplification?"

1. Administer a discrimination test at about 40-dB HL. This represents a level of soft conversational speech.
2. Administer some form of discrimination test at 70 to 80-dB HL (90 to 100 SPL). This is the level of loud conversational speech.
3. If the discrimination score is improved at 70 dB over that of 40 dB by at least 12%, one can assume that the subject can benefit from some form of amplification. This is not to say that the patient will be motivated to wear a hearing aid. It merely indicates that, all other things being equal, amplification can be of assistance.

DETERMINATION OF GAIN AND
MAXIMUM POWER OUTPUT REQUIREMENTS

Since gain is the electroacoustic characteristic designed to compensate for hearing loss, the amount and type of gain is of the utmost importance. Logic suggests that, if a person has a 50-dB hearing loss, the more gain that can be utilized to restore the functional acuity (aid of threshold to normal), the better the hearing aid fitting will be. However, this is not consistent with the physiological facts. It is a faulty assumption which has led to innumerable cases of overfitting in the past years.

Use-gain is 50% of Hearing Loss

My data suggest that the view held by many clinicians—that the more gain which can be utilized the better—may be faulty. Figure 3 illustrates the amount of use-gain as determined by 200 hearing aid users based on a comfort level setting. That is, it illustrates the gain actually being utilized at a comfort level setting as determined by the patient himself. It can be seen that the use-gain does not nearly approximate the amount of hearing loss. For example, the loss of 50-dB HL utilizes about 25-dB of gain and, as a general rule, will not tolerate more. Stated differently, a loss of 50-db HL (70 dB SPL) with an input speech signal of 60-dB SPL to the ear. This is a loud, but not intolerable, level. If, on the other hand, a person with a 50-dB loss were to attempt to utilize 50-dB of gain

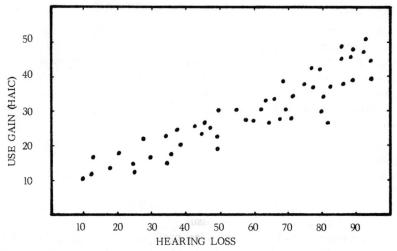

Figure 3. The average amount of use-gain at a comfort level setting in a group of 50 hearing aid users.

with a 60-dB input, the sound pressure at the ear would be 110 dB and would be unacceptable since the ear is overloaded. Virtually all speech, even conversational levels, would be annoying at this level. It can be seen that a general rule for use-gain is approximately 50% of the hearing loss determined by the average gain at 500, 1,000, and 2,000 Hz.

Other Tests

Other tests may be utilized in the selection procedure, that is, discrimination tests, tests of binaural-monaural function, etc. However, if excessive gain and maximum power output are presented exceeding the patient's threshold of discomfort, other tests become invalid as they preclude ultimate utilization and acceptance of the hearing aid. Stated differently, one can select an aid with a proper frequency response and having low distortion characteristics. However, if excessive gain and maximum power output is present, the most carefully selected hearing aid will likely be rejected.

SPECIAL CONSIDERATIONS
IN FITTING CHILDREN AND GERIATRIC PATIENTS

The purpose of this section of the paper is to illustrate some of the overlooked problems in fitting infants and children and to give suggestions in fitting procedures and adjustments of the aid.

Presbycusis

Somewhat over 60% of the patients with hearing aids are over 55 years of age. It is incumbent that the clinician, therefore, be aware of the various types of presbycusis. Each pathological type must be considered independently in evaluation of hearing aids. The following types of presbycusis have been identified:

Sensory Presbycusis Sensory presbycusis is characterized by changes in the supporting structures and hair cells in the cochlea.

Neural Presbycusis Neural presbycusis is characterized by the loss of ganglian cells and neurons, but may also involve neuronal cells in the brainstem.

Metabolic Presbycusis Metabolic presbycusis is characterized by changes, either within the cochlea or in the nerve tracts, causing specific or generalized degeneration of neural tissue.

Mechanical Presbycusis Mechanical presbycusis is caused by the aging process; a stiffening or other alteration of cells and other membranes may occur, resulting on altered function, especially within the cochlea.

Congenital Delayed Hearing Loss Congenital delayed hearing loss, a type of hearing loss beginning at middle age and slowly progressing, has been described. It is genetically determined, but becomes progressive, beginning at 30 to 50 years of age.

Central Degenerative Deafness Central degenerative deafness is characterized by loss of short-term memory, disorientation, and some forms of auditory discrimination problems. It is also characterized by delayed responses to auditory stimuli and increased time necessary for integration of auditory input.

Some of the above types of presbycusis are compatible to the introduction of hearing aids, whereas the chance of fitting other types is virtually zero.

SUGGESTED TESTS IN HEARING AID EVALUATION PROCEDURE

1. Careful case history: the clinician must determine what is the normal hearing loss expected for the patient's age. A hearing aid is not generally indicated in mild, high frequency losses, especially if it is within the expected norms of any age group.
2. Standard tests
   a. Aid conduction and bone conduction.
   b. Speech threshold and discrimination function up to 100-dB HL.
   c. The audiometric configuration.
3. Special tests
   a. Tests of recruitment: in the aging patient, the presence of recruitment is a positive sign suggesting that the lesion is in the cochlea and, contrary to popular belief, the aging patient with recruitment is one of the better candidates for a hearing aid.
   b. Tests for retrocochlear integrity: the administration of discrimination tests at comfortable level settings, at high intensities, and also the presence of tone decay, may suggest the presence of a retrocochlear lesion.
4. Tests of tolerance for dynamic range: this can be determined simply by determining the point which an individual *first* becomes annoyed at loud sounds. It is not the point at which the sound becomes painful. It is the point at which the sound first becomes uncomfortable or annoying since it is beyond this point that he will not tolerate sounds for any length of time.
5. Binaural integration and fusion: the ability to integrate sounds between the ears sometimes is suggestive of a brainstem or central lesion.

Table 1. Hearing aid fitting for the aging

Loss	Use-gain	Maximum gain	MPO	
			Loss	MPO
Cochlear (sensory)	½% average hearing loss	10–15 dB over the use-gain setting	20	95-dB SPL
			40	105-dB SPL
			60	115-dB SPL
			80	122-dB SPL
			100	130-dB SPL
Retrocochlear (neural)[a]	30–50% of average hearing loss, i.e., under fit for gain	10–15 dB over the use-gain settings		Usually 105–110 dB
Central auditory impairment	Less than 10% probability of successful hearing aid use			

[a]Be certain to test for reduction of discrimination while wearing the aid. If reduced 10% or more, aid may be contraindicated.

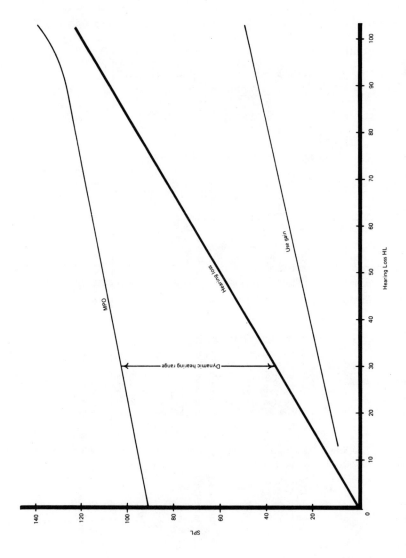

Figure 4. The recommended maximum power output and gain requirements as a function of hearing loss.

Table 2. Classifications of hearing impairment in children

Age	Classifications
Birth–5 months	1. Hearing normal or better than 60 dB 2. Severe to profound loss
6 months–1 year	1. Hearing normal or better than 45 dB 2. Moderate to severe loss (45–90 dB) 3. Profound loss (90 dB+)
1 year–3 years	1. Normal or mild loss (0–30 dB) 2. Moderate loss (45–60 dB) 3. Severe loss (60–90 dB) 4. Profound loss (90 dB+)
4 years–6 years	1. Normal (< 30 dB) 2. Mild loss (30–45 dB) 3. Moderate loss (45–60 dB) 4. Severe loss (60–90 dB) 5. Profound loss (90 dB+)

6. Response time: careful observation of the patient's response time to pure tone speech stimuli or conceptual questions containing conceptual constructs may be suggestive of a central type lesion.

HEARING AID FITTING FOR THE AGED

Table 1 gives an outline of suggested procedures in fitting the geriatric patient (see also Figure 4).

Table 3. Guide to be used to help select appropriate electroacoustic characteristics of the hearing aid

Loss	Use-gain	MPO	Frequency-response
Moderate (≤ 60 dB)	½ hearing loss	115-dB SPL (maximum)	Approximately 6 dB/octave rise
Severe (60–90 dB)	½ hearing loss	120 dB	Approximately 6 dB/octave rise
Profound (90 dB+)	50–60 dB	130–135 dB	Flat or low frequency

FITTING CHILDREN

Children with hearing loss differ from the geriatric population in that most have congenital hearing losses. The losses in more than 90% of the cases probably occur before or at the time of birth. Most children who come in for hearing aid evaluations will manifest a severe to profound loss since the mild losses are rarely detected at an early age.

Unique Fitting Problems of Children

A first step in evaluating children is to classify hearing loss. There are compromises in the accuracy of determining extent of loss; however, the following classifications can usually be made (Tables 2 and 3).

DISCUSSION

"BEST" FREQUENCY RESPONSE

AUDIENCE MEMBER: Even though an audiologist may prescribe a hearing aid, or adjust a hearing aid to a particular individual, if an electroacoustical measurement is not made on that particular hearing aid before it is recommended, the recommendation will be wrong because more than 50% of hearing aids do not have the frequency response shown in the specifications.

DR. McCANDLESS: Let me play the devil's advocate for a moment. What is right? In other words you mention prescribing a hearing aid. I just want to carry this a little further. What is right? What is the criteria for right? I do not know that. What is a right frequency response?

MR. VILLCHUR: Ah, my grandfather used to buy his glasses from a pushcart on the lower east side. That's right? I am sorry that that is the stage at which hearing aids are today, and that is the way we have to do it.

AUDIENCE MEMBER: You are asking the question, Dr. McCandless, but what do you actually do in fact? Do you do the best you can and prescribe, or do you describe what you think the hearing aid should have? Do you know what to do? You play the devil's advocate and you give a lot of negatives, but what do *you* do positively? How do you deal with the person who comes in with a hearing problem?

CRITICAL APPRAISAL OF
ELECTROACOUSTICAL CHARACTERITICS

DR. McCANDLESS: It is important for us to start taking another look at our priorities. In other words, what electroacoustic characteristics are important? What is the relative importance of the various electroacoustic characteristics that Mark Ross talks about? What are the relative important characteristics as far as the ear is concerned? Some of them can be thrown out completely. Some seem to retain a great deal of attention. Nonlinear amplification, for example, is very important because it is an attempt to compensate for the loudness distortion. That is one of the higher order priorities. Does it matter whether or not there is a +6 or a +3, or −2 slope? In order of priority, I would have to slip this down, based on available evidence. Let me ask a clinical question. How many times do audiologists talk about the recruiting ear and the gain characteristic and conclude that recruitment is characterized by reduced tolerance? How many think that if a patient has recruitment he has to have reduced tolerance? What evidence is there that that is true? I have evidence that it is not, but at least 50% of audiologists think it is true.

MEASUREMENT OF DYNAMIC RANGE

AUDIENCE MEMBER: Zenith did a report some time ago just on that question. They asked people to report how they measured the threshold of discomfort in hearing aid evaluations. Some used cold running speech in a hearing aid environment and established a tolerance level of 80 dB. Another used a recorded newscast by Fulton Lewis, Jr. Another said he kept going louder until the client grabbed the earphones from the ear or winced in pain. Again, the point was made. How can we possibly prescribe the electroacoustics, the compression, slope, recovery, overshoot, undershoot, transient distortion, and other characteristics when we do not have a measure that is reasonably acceptable that tells us about the dynamic range of the ear. It is sad.

USING A MASTER HEARING AID

AUDIENCE MEMBER: For the past few years I've done about 500 evaluations using a master hearing aid, which clinically works very well. Clinicians can look at the results on the master hearing aid and then shoot for best discrimination. This seems to be the best procedure under today's circumstances. Given the instruments on the market today, clinicians can do it so that the patient is satisfied. We can improve the discrimination scores of someone who is working with an aid, as much as 30 or 40%, and get some terrific results using the master hearing aid. If an aid does work, there is evidence to show it.
AUDIENCE MEMBER: I just bought a master hearing aid. For 2 years we have been using the Auricon and we switched to the Zenith one, which I like very much.

AUDIENCE MEMBER: How closely have you followed-up with patients? Have you seen them in 6 months to a year?

AUDIENCE MEMBER: We see them forthe original evaluation and then we send them for a trial period, and have them back in 3 to 4 weeks, which is the only time we really get them.

DR. ROSS: I have always found it a bit difficult to accept the idea that clinically audiologists work with somebody and say, "Hey, we helped this person who had this hearing loss; we put a hearing aid on him and helped him." For most people with a hearing loss, you can almost go to the pushcart and put something on and get some help, but the question we have to ask is, "How do we get the *most* help?" What is the ultimate? How far can we go with what particular electroacoustic measurement? What particular characteristic of hearing would produce the best type of response? We have to move away from the pushcart.

NARROW BAND NOISE AS A TEST STIMULUS

AUDIENCE MEMBER: We are dealing with two slightly separate problems. One is the patient who has speech and language and an acquired hearing loss through age or noise or whatever. The second is the child who has to be fitted and does not have speech and language. I do not have a master hearing aid, but I have a lot of hearing aids at my disposal. I test adults totally differently from the way I test children.

I test the children with narrow band noise. How do you account for the fact that a hearing aid which amplifies up to 4,300 Hz will elicit a response at 8,000 Hz to narrow band noise in the sound field?

DR. ROSS: What is the skirt of the noise? Some of these third octave filters have a very wide skirt.

AUDIENCE MEMBER: How do I know that, with the narrow band noise I am generating, the child is getting enough amplification to produce intelligible speech?

DR. ROSS: I gather you mean a preverbal hearing-impaired child.

HEARING AID SELECTION FOR THE PRE-VERBAL CHILD

AUDIENCE MEMBER: In a recent article I read that recorded conversational speech was related to a contour of narrow band noise. That was the input level. The child was tested in the sound field with the narrow band noise to find threshold and after that the child was tested again with narrow band noise using a hearing aid. What the study did was to try to find a tolerance level, noting that all a child needed was perhaps 10 dB or 20 dB above threshold to get enough sound for intelligible speech. They concluded that the aid should supply the best sensation level across frequency because, with the pre-verbal child, they couldn't predict how much intelligible speech the child was going to get. The only way to do it was to use a reference point from regular conversational speech to aided sensation levels.

DR. ROSS: That was the Central Institute for the Deaf group study. I finished a chapter on, "Hearing Aid Selection with Pre-Verbal Children," in which I discussed the sound pressure level method. It seems right. What has to be dealt with are the important cues in terms of the acoustics of speech. The electroacoustics of the hearing aid and the characteristics of the ear both help determine what the perceived sensation levels would be across frequencies. These factors would predict what is potentially audible and potentially available to the children. Given the limitations of what we know, we know more than we currently use.

EAR-LEVEL VERSUS BODY-WORN AMPLIFICATION

DR. McCANDLESS: This is precisely what we found: use-gain is almost proportional to the hearing loss. The person with the 60 dB loss would use almost exactly 30 dB of gain. There is some variance, depending upon the slope, but the average of the best two frequencies is very, very close, because it is related to loudness. For example, 90 dB losses average about 40 to 45 dB use-gain. Why do we then have body aids on 90 dB losses if the patients are using 40 dB of gain? In other words, unless patients are using vibrotactile stimulation, as far as we are concerned, body aids just are not needed.

DR. ROSS: I agree with you, but there are other reasons.

DR. McCANDLESS: Yes—with children.

DR. ROSS: The durability of body aids is one reason, but even that is not a good one. Until quite recently, the other reason was that ear-level aids did not provide a wide enough band width.

METHODS OF PLOTTING USE-GAIN

DR. McCANDLESS: Yes, that is another reason. We then tried to take a retrospective look and see what was happening in real life and construct a procedure on that basis. We simply took this use-gain figure and found the variance. We could go back and predict the use-gain and set it within 1 dB of what a patient would set it at using the acoustic reflex measure, the beginning acoustic reflex. That is one way, but, if you do not have the acoustic reflex, you have to use something else.

For children, we simply took the hearing loss and plotted the use-gain based on thousands of measures. The variance of this gain is going to be less than ±3 or 4 dB and the overload is going to be about ±4 dB. We can go to the chart, look at the hearing loss, and plot the maximum power output and the use-gain, again, retrospectively. There are some other variables, but at least this is one way. We have done this arbitrarily now on 200 consecutive patients. We can do it in 15 minutes, and what has happened is that we have reduced the rejection rate to virtually 0. Losses of 70 dB require less than 120 dB output. We have been overfitting universally.

AUDIENCE MEMBER: What stimulus do you use to elicit the reflex?

DR. McCANDLESS: Narrow band noise will be fine. Speech is probably the best.

AUDIENCE MEMBER: Have you checked any conductive cases or are they too rare?

USE-GAIN AND MPO FOR CONDUCTIVE LOSSES

DR. McCANDLESS: Conductive losses will have an altogether different dynamic range. Their MPOs won't be quite as high as normal. You can't count on most conductive losses unless they have an acute case of otitis media, where there is some pain involved. You can probably go to maximum of 130 to 135 dB with no trouble. The above only applies to conductive lesions.

OVERFITTING BY THE PATIENT

MR. VILLCHUR: Overfitting is even worse because one of the persons that does the overfitting is the patient. Since the patient wants to hear the weak consonants that he is unable to hear, he turns his gain control up so that he can still tolerate the sound but the loud sounds, the vowels, are really louder than he wants in order to make it possible for him to hear the consonants. Every one of my six subjects, when he went to the compression mode of amplification, chose to listen at a reduced average level, although the level of the weak portions of the sound at which he was actually listening was increased.

DR. ROSS: You didn't stress one thing that you did and that was the equalization aspect. You did mention the high frequency emphasis, but actually didn't you parallel that equal-loudness contour in your delivered speech signal?

EQUAL-LOUDNESS CONTOUR
PARALLELS PREFERRED SPEECH LEVELS

MR. VILLCHUR: Yes, this was a laboratory situation and I matched very carefully. I was using a multifilter and I could adjust each adjacent third octave band, but this is not practical in a real hearing aid.

I wonder what audiologists do if things are so terrible? What do you do with the real patient that comes in? What would I do in terms of what is available today?

In my study, the subject was measured in the laboratory. I had his threshold and I had his equal-loudness contour measured in the third octave intervals. I want to point out that what was seen in the laboratory was typical. The equal-loudness contour measured at the preferred speech level tended to follow the general curve of the threshold, but at a much reduced slope and with much reduced peaks and troughs. Typically, the curve would be flatter than that, with an even greater flattening out of the peaks and troughs of the threshold. Our procedure was as follows: we measured the patient's threshold and his preferred speech level (the level at which he would rather listen to speech). Suppose we found he liked to listen to the speech sample at about 20 dB higher than a normal person would. Then we had some idea whether to use a compressor hearing aid, the amount of compression that he needed, and we certainly had some idea of the general slope of the frequency response that he was likely to find useful. It gave us a general direction. After that we tried three or four aids, but we could choose them on the basis of their characteristics.

BACKWARD AND FORWARD MASKING

Another factor was the problem of forward masking. That is a phenomenon in which a loud vowel tends to mask the succeeding consonant, and it is very faint. About 20 years ago, experimenters found that introducing a severe low frequency cut into reception improved intelligibility considerably. The majority of hearing aids on the market today provide something of the order of 18 dB per octave attenuation below about 700 Hz. Sometimes this is useful and sometimes it is not. There are some hearing aids which provide a relatively flat response down to the lower frequencies. It is important to know which of the two aids is being used. This can be determined purely on the basis of a behavioral test. It doesn't seem to follow the normal rules, and I suspect that that is because there is no easy test for the relative importance of the low frequencies.

RELATION OF
ELECTROACOUSTICAL FACTORS TO PERFORMANCE

DR. WHITE: In our work, we believe that first one should study the operation of the ear and then try and relate electroacoustic characteristics to the needs that appear. What we are trying to do is to fall somewhere between those two extremes. We are not strongly interested in acoustic characteristics. I happen to be, but that is not the area that we will be spending a lot of time on. We have a master hearing aid that is, in a sense, some kind of a black box, and what we are trying to develop is a procedure that will explore many possible settings to help some ears. We have an experimental design that does this and then permits us to look afterward at the acoustic characteristics.

MASTER HEARING AID AND
AUDITORY TRAINING AS PART OF THE SELECTION PROCESS

AUDIENCE MEMBER: We have talked about better knowledge and understanding of the electroacoustic characteristics and their use. We talked about better diagnostic procedures. The one thing that we have not talked about too much, which the Master Hearing Aid Study is incorporating, is the entire selection paradigm itself. Many audiologists tend to feel they can take one test session, or one test, and find out which is the best hearing aid, if they are using very sophisticated methodology. A very important aspect is spreading out the selection process by using auditory training or therapy. Then, a hearing aid selection can be made on the basis of how a person does over a prolonged period of time using a master hearing aid perhaps, but it should be tried with auditory therapy. Nobody is going to put on a hearing aid and do as well during that session as he would perhaps 1 week later. His brain has had time to adjust. That is an important part and, in Tennessee, audiologists are doing that. The idea is to fit hearing aids on a patient after a long period of selection based on how the person performs during auditory therapy with a master hearing aid.

HOSPITAL CLINICS VERSUS UNIVERSITY CLINICS

AUDIENCE MEMBER: That's great if audiologists can get people to do it. How in the world do you get somebody to do it in a hospital that says, "You have this many dollars to make this week in order to keep yourself in this job." That is what it really comes down to in the long run. If an audiologist sees one person for 1 hour and five people that day, and the same people will be seen the next week, then they have to be charged $15 an hour. They are not going to come back! What can be done in a university clinic is very different from what can be done in a hospital.

MASTER HEARING AID PROGRAMMING

AUDIENCE MEMBER: That's for sure, the real world compared to the other. What information does Dick White put into a master hearing aid? What is the criteria for selecting beginning points in this black box with different choices?

DR. WHITE: What we try to do is gain from two approaches. Our design incorporated various fixed choices of hearing aid configurations. The general idea is to test the aid set in those ways with everybody. In other words, no judgments. Certain choices do not work and certain of them do. It is not always what one expects. Starting from those points, audiologists would use their own insights into ways to change them. What we did was to try to do an investigation first that would be as little biased as possible by people's preconception.

MPO LIMITERS AND OVERLOAD

AUDIENCE MEMBER TO DR. McCANDLESS: People on your charts with quite a bit of hearing loss seem to require very low maximum power output. Where do you set your maximum power output in the cases you talked about, and what kind of power limiters do you use?

DR. McCANDLESS: The most significant finding of our work corresponds with some of the work of others. My entire concept of the upward usable hearing range was in error for me. What the books say is that a person with normal or pathological ear can hear and understand sound pressures in excess of 100 dB, which is true. We can hear and we can discriminate clear up to 140, but the question is, "Is 140 dB, therefore, the sensible upper usable hearing range?" We know what the minimum is, we know what the frequency extensions are, but what is overload; what is too much? This is the question we addressed ourselves to. As an aside, compression years ago was originally designed to avoid *that* complaint—the loud sounds from coming in so abruptly. Actually, the work that Ed Villchur was talking about and maximum power output are two separate issues. In other words, we compress to compensate for the recruitment phenomenon and we shape the curve, which is great. Completely separate, and perhaps even a different mechanism, is this question of *too much.* These should be considered as two separate questions.

"HOW MUCH IS TOO MUCH MPO?"

DR. McCANDLESS: Getting back then to the issue of how much is too much, we did two things. We asked people to let us know when it was too much. We also took a different approach and simply said, "How much are you using? How much do you want?" We did not find one patient, and we still have not found any one patient with acoustic reflexes, who, with the hearing aid on, would allow us simply to go on and on indefinitely. People just will not do it. Secondly, the point of beginning discomfort is like saying, "I am going to give you a shot—tell me when you can't stand it any longer." Some people will yell as soon as it is a foot away. Other people could be jabbed all day. What is the magic number? It depends on one's criteria. We can change the instructions, or we can actually find out what people are experiencing, which is what we did, and we found that it was much lower than we had ever suspected. It did not coincide with Davis and Silverman's estimate of 130 dB for everybody, but it is near 95 or even 90 for many, many people with mild losses.

MPO PREDICTIVE CHARTS

We plotted this function to find exactly what output level should be and to develop charts on the basis of a predictive value. Based on those charts we know what the deviation is and use hearing aids with those characteristics to boil it down to one or two in 5 minutes. The upper level is lower than we ever suspected. There is a different criterion involved, and it has a physiological base. There is a mechanism which says "too much," and Hood and Poole's data suggested this clearly. If it is 5 dB over this level, then it is beginning to be too much, and drastic temporary threshold shifts will result. Physiological changes do occur.
AUDIENCE MEMBER: Are you fitting hearing aids with a maximum power output in that range?

TURNING GAIN DOWN BECAUSE OF OVERLOAD

DR. McCANDLESS: Yes. If it is in excess of this psychophysiological limit, people will turn down the gain to compensate. Ed Villchur mentioned this. They will simply turn down the gain to cut the maximum power output down.

GAIN AND MPO FOR THE PROFOUNDLY DEAF

DR. ROSS: Sometimes we are in a position of nine blind men and the elephant. We all describe the animal differently, depending on the portion of the anatomy that we feel. Myself, if I see a kid with a 50-dB loss, or a 60-dB loss or less, he's almost like a godsend. Where did this easy case come from? In a school for the deaf, we deal with 90- and 100-dB losses all the time! We are dealing with a different order of being.

DR. McCANDLESS: This is a very important point. Why is it then that some kids with severe and profound losses will turn up their gain and let the aid squeal all day, if what I said is true? The answer to that is a very simple one. Again, it is physiologically based. If one has sufficient sensory reserve to achieve a certain amount of loudness, this discomfort level is real. It corresponds with the reflex when it is present and it is very consistent. However, if one does not have sufficient sensory units to elicit this reflex action, that something up here says "too much," then one does not get the same sensation, and this discomfort level is bypassed completely. In those cases, aids can be used which will go up to 130 to 140 dB. It is easy to find out. It is a test that we now have. In those cases, power is wanted, but only in those cases.

LEVEL OF DISCOMFORT
DOES NOT CHANGE AFTER HEARING AID USE

AUDIENCE MEMBER: Don't people learn to use and normalize the sound they consistently experience?

DR. McCANDLESS: That is an interesting question. Since we are dealing with old wives' tales, I was taught that if you put a hearing aid on a person they would learn to tolerate it. Now, I just can't, in good conscience, buy that concept. It is true that people adapt. As the gentleman said, "They learn to incorporate more things over time." That is true. But, does anything change physiologically? The answer, at least with our data, is absolutely not. We have evaluated people in whom this is unchanged over a period of 7 years. As a matter of fact, the discomfort level will go down. How many times do we find the comfort level—and patients come back with the aid turned down, not up? In 98% of the subjects tested, the preferred listening level was down after the first test, not up, which gives credence to my comments about this physiological level.

PATIENT'S CONTRIBUTION TO HEARING AID LEVEL

MR. VILLCHUR: I worked with the same subjects for as long as a year and started out with two misconceptions, both of which I quickly had to disabuse myself. One was that I knew better than the subjects what was good for them. I would adjust all the dials so that my speech band fit beautifully in between the threshold and the equal loudness contour which was carefully measured, and so forth, and then I would ask them to touch up the dials until the thing sounded best to them. They would always change it somewhat. In some cases, I had hit fairly closely, but, in some cases, they would change it quite a bit, and I gave them a lot of choices. Then I tested them, without their knowing what was happening, of course, both at my settings and at their settings. When they came back the next time, I would carefully deceive them by unloosening the set screws on the knob, moving them so that the pointer was in a different direction, and say, "I want to check it. Please would you set the dials again?" They would end up with totally different numbers, but they were consistently right. In other words, their settings gave them higher scores than mine did, and, furthermore, in order not to confuse the idea of pleasantness of the sound and intelligibility, there were cases where they would say, "Well, this set of characteristics is more intelligible than this set of characteristics, but *less* pleasant." The ultimate set of characteristics *always* gave higher intelligibility and either equal or better index of pleasantness or comfort.

The other procedure I had to stop was doing the opposite. I said, "Please, *you* set all the dials." They were lost. Clinicians have got to put them in the ball park because there are too many interrelated characteristics, and, if one gets set wrong, then the other will never get to the right place. The only way that I could get the answers was to put them in the right ball park by intuition or calculation and then let them readjust in some kind of a rational order.

MOST COMFORTABLE LOUDNESS LEVEL MEASUREMENT

AUDIENCE MEMBER: I have been using narrow band noise to find a most comfortable level. What is the most comfortable level slope across frequencies, say from 500 to 4,000, that an audiologist should test for, and what is its implication for discrimination? I'm working with severely and profoundly hard of hearing college-age students and I've been keeping track of the slopes measured.

I have also been measuring the uncomfortable levels of students across frequencies and found more problems at 1,000 Hz than at any of the other frequencies. Have any other people found the same effects?

MR. VILLCHUR: I would have confidence in a most comfortable level curve if it did what the equal loudness curve did. In other words, if it appeared to follow the general shape of the threshold curve but at reduced slope and at reduced distance between peaks and troughs. That's what I would expect. That does not mean that it would be so in every case, but, generally, that would be the thing to look for.

VALIDATING THE MOST COMFORTABLE LEVEL OF LOUDNESS

DR. ROSS: We can determine most comfortable level and uncomfortable level, but there has been enough suggestion that audiologists have been doing some things which should be changed. That worries me. One way we can develop a little security in what we are doing is to think again about the validation procedure—and that is to get back to the old problem of how do we validate in terms of speech discrimination? Shouldn't we validate the most-comfortable-level and uncomfortable-level measures by considering how the person listens or hears with that setting out in the environment?

IS THE BODY HEARING AID OBSOLETE?

AUDIENCE MEMBER: May we have further comment on whether the body aid is obsolete for somebody with a 90-dB hearing loss? Can we expect to look forward to a future where postauricular aids are used on profoundly deaf children as a routine thing, while body aids will be used only if something special is needed.

DR. ROSS: In my school (The Willie Ross School for the Deaf), my last older child is getting ear-level aids next week. Many of my younger ones still have body aids. I have been interested for a long time in frequencies past 3,000 Hz and have found it inconceivable and unjustifiable to put aids on children omitting the spectral information past 3,000 Hz which conveys possessive information, pluralization information, as well as phonological information. Until recently, ear-level aids have not done that, but now, with some ear-level aids, you *can* go up to 5,000 and 6,000 Hz.

To answer your point, as far as children are concerned, the idea was that you can put an ear-level aid on a child, but it will be broken the next week. Therefore, you can't do it because he will break it every week! I'd rather try first—I think the ear-level location is 100% better.

People ask me, "Okay, what are you doing wearing that aid on *your* body?" There are two reasons. First of all, I get my aids from the Veterans Administration. The other reason is, if a person has a fairly stiff eardrum, a drum with a high impedance characteristic caused by either lesions or fluid, he will get feedback at a usage level where he does not ordinarily have feedback with a button receiver. I don't get feedback when I put the aid in my pocket, but if I put it right by my ear where I would ordinarily locate it, I get feedback. A lot of energy is being reflected off the drum and picked up by the microphone and amplified. There is some evidence, at least in terms of a good, nice, compliant drum, that one can attenuate at least 50 dB from the tip of the earmold to the microphone without feedback. That is the average, nice ear drum with nice compliance attributes. For some of these children who have chewed up ear drums, that may not be true.

AUDIENCE MEMBER: Everybody seems to be condemning body aids because they have too much maximum power output, but there are body hearing aids that have much lower acoustic output than postauricular aids. There are a lot of geriatric people I work with on whom I would not dream of putting behind-the-ear aids, especially some Parkinson cases. The hearing aid is going to fall off before the patient even gets near it!

DR. ROSS: That is right. There are different indications for an elderly person with palsy also.

EFFECT OF AMBIENT NOISE ON SPEECH RECEPTION

AUDIENCE MEMBER: Why do some people who get very poor discrimination scores with amplification function very well under phones?

DR. ROSS: I have a record that will illustrate that. With a telephone, you have a nice signal. You can put that thing right on your ear and you can block out all the noise. You've got a hearing aid 6, 8, or 10 feet away from the speech and you get a poor signal. That is a simple explanation. There is also a difference in monosyllabic discrimination and sentence discrimination.

MR. VILLCHUR: The additional advantage of the telephone is lack of reverberation. The mouthpiece is less than an inch away from the speaker's mouth and all the room noise is kept out.

AUDIENCE MEMBER: If someone is talking on the phone, he probably knows what the conversation is about, whereas, with giving monosyllabic words, people do not know what to expect. A study was done with air traffic controllers and background noise, and the investigators tried to demonstrate the degree to which they could reduce the speech signal and still have the air controller understand. They found that speech could be reduced immensely and controllers could understand because controllers only had 2,000 words in their technical vocabulary.

DR. ROSS: There is a nice relationship between a restriction of a discrimination set and the signal and noise relationship with which you can understand the set. The more you can predict the language, the poorer the signal-to-noise relationship can be.

AUDIENCE MEMBER: There is a lot of difference between aids in understanding on the telephone. Sometimes I choose the aid on how well the child understands me through the phone.

DR. ROSS: Categorical thinking of any kind is what we have to fear. We all do categorical thinking; the body versus ear-level categorical thinking; oral-manual categorical thinking. We are dealing with interactions of personal physiological characteristics, hearing aid characteristics, identification characteristics. I won't mention them all, but all of them must be considered.

DR. WHITE: Since people have been making this distinction between postauricular and body aids, our unit is essentially a postauricular aid. It has two wires coming out of it—one for the receiver to the microphone. In a sense, we are getting the best of both worlds. The unit is flexible and easy to handle, but the microphone is placed in a good position on the head.

DR. ROSS: I have an ideal aid which I have asked companies to make, but it has never come true. If they could take White's unit (which is really a binaural ear-level hearing aid) and include FM receiver capability, then the same unit could be worn at home and in school, in and out of class, and individual and group instruction. That was my dream.

REAL EAR-AIDED MEASUREMENTS

DR. WHITE: At all stages through our tests, we measure narrow band noise hearing thresholds in the sound-field situation. We measure this with someone both wearing a hearing aid and not. The point is presumably that the difference between the curves with and without a hearing aid tells something about the effective gain or the effective frequency response of that hearing aid on somebody's ear. It may have a strong correlation with the kind of measurements you would make with a probe microphone. The reason for doing this is that it tells the audiologist what the functional gain of the aid is rather than the gain which may be measured artifically in a

2-cc coupler. This measurement will give us a way of explaining otherwise inexplicable results.

AUDIENCE MEMBER: I have been doing that with children, as well as with anybody that just does not have good speech. The problem that I have found with the comparison of aided versus unaided thresholds is the practical problem of trying to explain to the parent why I am doing that measurement. I try to show parents that their child can hear better with a particular aid. I can tell in my audiologist's jargon, and be as basic as possible, why one aid is better, and the parent still says, "I was tested here 3 years ago and that is not what 'they' said." Those are the kinds of problems we face.

DR. WHITE: Yes, that is a good point, and we are very lucky because we are choosing people who tend to be unhappy with hearing aids. We are able, at least in the initial stages, to pay them for their listening time. That is a different thing. We are spending a lot of testing time, more than would be reasonable to spend in a clinic, because we do not know too well what we are going to end up with or what we are looking for. For that reason, we have to give participants some kind of recompense.

CHOOSING THE BEST HEARING AID

DR. McCANDLESS: Somebody asked a question related to the more practical aspects of fitting and selection. Do we really want to say that one aid is best? Either the patient said, "I'll take this one and this one" or the audiologist said, "These are the aids I think the patient wants and I'll let him try them." I do not know what the criterion for such a choice would be. You mentioned validation. One method of validation is not rejection. If they do not put it in a drawer, you are a success.

HEARING AIDS SHOULD BE DEFINED IN OPERATIONAL TERMS

DR. ROSS: That takes us back to another interesting point. We have always talked about one aid versus another aid or about body aids versus ear-level aids. We really should be talking about what this aid does. There are conveniences which are aspects of ear-level and body aids in terms of location, microphone, and clothing noise. There are also presumably describable differences in the performance of the aid to which we can attribute some of the differences. If a body aid does better, it does better for a reason and I would want to know what the reason is. The reason should be describable in terms we can understand.

MR. VILLCHUR: It may not be because it is a body aid.

HEARING AIDS FOR INFANTS AND CHILDREN

DR. McCANDLESS: How can we, in the fitting of children, correlate the incomplete test results which we have with the need to put on amplification? The following paradigm was developed as a result of the work of several clinics. Most of us feel fairly comfortable with a general classification of hearing between the ages of birth and 5 months as being normal or better than 60 dB, or as being a severely profound loss. We hope we can do better, but we can at least do this much. By 6 months to 1 year, we can usually make at least three general categorizations: normal hearing or better than 45 dB, moderate to severe hearing loss, or profound loss. We can do this relatively easily. At about 1 to 3 years, we can generally make four classifications normal, mild, moderate, or profound. Our distinctions are usually not much finer than that. By 4 to 6 years, we can make a precise categorization. We feel badly that we cannot make these five categorizations at age 2 months because that would be a more reasonable testing paradigm.

What can we do as far as hearing aid fittings with this information? How do we select the characteristics, type of aid, or anything else on a child when we only know whether they have a hearing loss of 60 dB or better or 60 dB and worse. That is precisely the practical question with which we are confronted. If we want to fit children younger than 1 year, we can't be much more precise than this. We can say something generally about slope and maximum power output, but not much. How do we pick which ear? If a child has a loss less then 60 dB, set the gain to approximately one-half the hearing loss and it will be close. The maximal power output should not exceed 115 dB if it is less than 60 dB. Follow that scale up and we are right there.

As a general rule, the procedure is to choose an aid that has some low frequency attenuation. I would go along with the early Hudgins report. Even if the child had a severe loss, using these kinds of classifications, the use-gain is simply half the loss. Here again, one can go up to 120 dB maximum. Again, do the same thing for a flat loss. Use 50 to 60 dB of gain and an MPO of 100 to 135. We can categorize maximum power output and frequency response estimations based on whatever child classifications we have. Any time there is more than about a 10-dB per octave change in the frequency response, use the average of the two frequencies that have the most gain.

HEARING AID USE AT HALF VOLUME

AUDIENCE MEMBER: What about the use of hearing aid at one-half volume? Can you measure that? How does the frequency response differ?

DR. McCANDLESS: The frequency response, if it is fairly linear, unless there is overloading, shouldn't change that much. This is a suggestion. If a person has a 60-dB loss, he is going to be using about 25- to 30-dB gain. Add 10 or 15 fudge factor and one has peak gain, use-gain, and maximum power output all figured out as a ball park. Then an audiologist can do the kinds of things that Ed Villchur discussed in the juggling of precision. It can't be done on children, of course. As far as adults are concerned, many kinds of presbyacusics should be tested out beforehand. If the loss is sensory, then again, the use-gain is going to be approximately one-half, and the maximum gain is only going to be 10 to 15 dB over the use-gain setting. This is almost universal. This won't vary more than a couple of decibels. Check the table in the Appendix. For a 20-dB loss, it is going to be 105; 40-dB loss is going to be 107 or 108; 80-dB loss is only going to be about 120. If the loss is retrocochlear and, in addition, there is a sensory or cochlear impairment, then the hearing aid fitting will be altogether different.

ROLL-OVER PHENOMENON IN DISCRIMINATION TESTING

AUDIENCE MEMBER: Under the neural category, is discrimination reduced 10% or more?

DR. McCANDLESS: If a hearing aid is used and discrimination goes down regardless of modification, a roll-over phenomenon is indicated. Ten percent is fairly conservative, but on the other hand, why use an aid if it drops discrimination?

AUDIENCE MEMBER: I would not know if that was actually an accurate assessment of that person's discrimination. I would hate to see a decision based just on that.

DR. McCANDLESS: The thing to do in these cases is to do a roll-over function. Find out whether or not, at 100 dB, a reduction of discrimination is found. Do a PB function and find out.

ESSENTIALS OF A COMPLETE HEARING EVALUATION

DR. ROSS: It seems to me that the first part of the hearing aid evaluation has been minimized. Imagine doing a really complete audiological evaluation! By a really complete audiological evaluation, I mean building into audiometers a number of variable pass-band filters, electronic switches for controlling time, a variety of reverberation possibilities, interruption rate, and so on. A year ago, I tested pitch discrimination, and found people who literally could not tell the difference between a 1,000-cycle tone and a 4,000-cycle tone. These are the kinds of things which will have an effect upon how people are going to function with a hearing aid. If anyone thinks of a hearing aid evaluation as a one-shot affair, whether with a child or an adult, that child or adult will suffer. We cannot possibly predict performance after just one or two evaluations. Hearing aid evaluations, whether for children or adults, have to be considered part of a complete rehabilitation program. Some people will need more services, and some less. This has to be evaluated also. To draw upon the analogy I used earlier, we have to consider the whole elephant and not view any part of it as the whole creature.

SUMMARY
AND REVIEW

Mark Ross

We started out from different viewpoints, then seemed to converge, and wound up thinking about hearing aids and how to fit them.

REVIEW OF DR. ROSS' PRESENTATION

I presented the view that we have been talking about—hearing aid A versus hearing aid B, and hearing aid evaluation procedures, when we should be talking about electroacoustic system A versus electroacoustic system B. Then it is not a question of what one names an aid, but what it does that is important. We have been mislead somewhat in current hearing aid evaluation procedures by thinking we are evaluating different hearing aids when we are really evaluating different specific electroacoustic systems. Many hearing aids—any *one* hearing aid now—can replicate a number of amplification patterns. That was my basic thrust, and I supported it with some research which pointed out the importance of various dimensions of electroacoustic response to intelligibility. I also commented about current hearing aid evaluation procedures.

REVIEW OF MR. VILLCHUR'S PRESENTATION

Mr. Villchur, from the Foundation for Hearing Research of Woodstock, described the subjective sensation of a hearing-impaired listener with a high frequency loss and then corrected this—first by compression alone, then by high frequency emphasis alone, and then by the two in combination. He described this sensation without background noise and then with some background competing signals. The transformation in the intelligibility of the signal was quite impressive. His basic suggestion for signal processing was very attractive and has a great deal of merit in the future of hearing aid selection procedures.

Basically, what he did was to compress a signal and plot the auditory responses on a sound pressure level scale rather than on an audiogram. He plotted an equal-loudness contour on the same scale, looked at the acoustics of a speech signal on the same scale, and then compressed the signal. The signal was two bands, a low band and a high band, with some overlap in the middle. He then took the output of this compressed signal level, after checking the recruitment characteristics of the individual ear, and put it through a multifilter circuit which, in a sense, closely followed the contour of the equal-loudness line. He presented some impressive research results and a way of processing and packaging speech signals into the impaired listener's ear by compensating, not just for frequency, which is what has been done for years, but also for amplitude.

REVIEW OF DR. McCANDLESS PRESENTATION

The last speaker was Geary McCandless, of the University of Utah. Geary covered the ground and highlighted it again: the importance of really doing a careful audiological workup and looking at the characteristics of the impaired ear, which, after all, is where the packaged or processed signal will be delivered. He presented examples of the different effects resulting from pathology in the end organ, the hair cell, and the spiral ganglion. In one example, the patient had practically no cochlea at all because the cochlea ducts were filled with bone as in cases of congenital syphilis. He showed how all of these particular cases would have similar pure tone thresholds, but that the way in which they would discriminate a speech singal would be different. The level at which they would respond to a speech signal would further differentiate them. He described an example of loudness decay at high sound pressure levels, at a point where the normal listener could hold on to the loudness of a 110-dB sound for a fairly long period of time while the pathological listener would exhibit a rapid decay of the sound. This phenomenon, McCandless felt, had to have some effect on how an impaired listener processed speech.

The other major point that Dr. McCandless made, and further elaborated on, was something everyone said—"We tend to overfit patients in terms of gain and we tend to overfit them in terms of output." He presented some data where he plotted, on a single chart, the threshold responses, suggested gain, and suggested output, which were based on empirical data collected in over 200 cases. He analyzed the use-gain of instruments and related it to the hearing level of the patient, and found, as others in Europe have found, that the actual use-gain is somewhere around 50% of the hearing level. It has been a fairly typical and unfortunate procedure in audiology centers to try to compensate the degree of the loss by the amplification of the instrument. If somebody had a 70-dB loss, the audiologist used to think about an aid with 70 dB of gain. That was a poor example of clinic procedure. McCandless empirical data showed that actual use-gain is about 50%. The actual MPO should be based on the level of stapedial reflex elicitation. Audiologists should make more use of this objective measure in terms of setting output for a number of their patients.

The discussion that followed clarified these major presentations.

GENERAL
ASSEMBLY

DISCUSSION

Mark Ross, Chairman

PANEL CORRECTIONS: HIGH FREQUENCY AVERAGE

DR. SINCLAIR: I want to clear up one point on the high frequency average as it was mentioned. Manufacturers are not trying to emphasize high frequencies by picking new averages. The intent of getting a new frequency average is to match the measurements of the National Bureau of Standards. These three discrete frequencies came closest to matching their noise technique. We are not emphasizing high frequencies. We had to pick three new frequencies to match a noise technique which we could not duplicate in all the industry facilities, but we can duplicate in pure tone measurements. It will enable us to do that.

LABELING MPO

DR. WILBER: In light of one of the comments that was made in another group concerned about noise and high level gain instruments, we were pleased to learn that one of the standard suggestions was that, among new hearing aids, any aid that has an MPO of 132 dB will be so marked. It will clearly be apparent that that aid has an MPO of 132 dB.

DR. SINCLAIR: Yes, the FDA is pressing for that rule for *any* output over 130 dB. The aids will be labeled, or at least the material that goes with the aid will be clearly labeled, in words if it is over 132 dB.

AUDIOLOGISTS DISPENSING AIDS

DR. HARDICK: While we are correcting, Dr. Harris quoted me as saying that audiologists should take more of a leadership role in the dispensing of hearing aids and we should all work to upgrade the hearing aid dealer.

Without telling you what I would have said if asked, I can say that I made no such statement about the hearing aid dealer.

LOANER PROGRAMS FOR CHILDREN

DR. MADELL: I would like to correct an impression that came out of this morning's program. When talking about choosing hearing aids for very young children, I said that, before we choose a hearing aid, the child should have a long enough period to adjust to amplification so that a reasonable judgment about differences between hearing aid performance can be made. For a child with a profound hearing loss, it may take time before that kind of judgment can be made. Once the child has adjusted to amplification, however, the choice of a particular hearing aid can be made in a period of no more than a month—not several months.

USE-GAIN AND EQUAL-LOUDNESS CONTOURS

MR. VILLCHUR: May I comment instead about a confirmation? Mark Ross and Geary McCandless referred to the phenomenon of the actual use-gain of a hearing aid being on the order of $33\frac{1}{3}$ to 50% in terms of decibels of the hearing loss. One of the figures in my presentation bore that out rather well. There were four curves plotted: normal hearing threshold, the normal 74-phon equal-loudness contour which intersects the conversational speech band at 1 KHz, the abnormal threshold of a particular subject plotted at his preferred speech level. If the hearing loss is taken as the difference between normal threshold and his threshold, it was of the order of 1 KHz of 50 or 60 dB. If the hearing loss was taken as the difference between the normal equal-loudness contour and his equal-loudness contour at an equivalent speech level (which is also hearing loss, except it is not our conventional definition), it turned out that his hearing loss was indeed only 15 or 20 dB. This phenomenon about which Ross and McCandless spoke occurs because we conventionally define hearing loss as the loss at threshold. If we defined hearing loss in terms of the loss at conversational level, the actual loss would be far less and would more or less correspond to the use-gain concept.

DR. ROSS: Annette Zaner and Don Markle did a study where they developed a preferred "most comfortable loudness" in hearing aid selection. It may not be used very much clinically, but it certainly should be. We should consider the average input with a speech signal of about 65-dB SPL at 1,000 Hz where the most comfortable loudness again in sound pressure level terms is at 90 dB. Gain should be at that point which is at 25 dB. Looking at the difference between input and most comfortable loudness will provide a good idea of where to set the gain of the hearing aid. All of us have touched on this particular item. We are all thinking in terms of how to proceed in this area.

STANDARDIZED TESTS FOR CHILDREN

DR. GARDINER (AUDIENCE MEMBER): What standardized tests can be used with children to determine the best hearing aid?

DR. MADELL: Pure tones are one measure that one would use in doing hearing aid evaluations for children, but pure tone information is not enough. Tones are not discriminated with the same side of the brain. If the goal is that children should understand speech with their hearing aids, then we would like to measure speech. Dr. Ross has developed an excellent speech discrimination test, the Word Intelligibility by Picture Identification Test, which we use regularly with children with profound hearing losses, but the child needs to have some language. If the child does not have sufficient language to use a test like the WIPI, we ask the child's speech and hearing clinician to provide us with a list of words that the child can discriminate using auditory signals alone. Either the clinician provides pictures or we provide our own pictures, and we use a nonstandard discrimination test. This can be a very valuable tool in evaluating the child's ability to discriminate. We also use the standard W22 lists on many children, even those with profound losses.

TESTS FOR THE PRE-VERBAL CHILD

DR. ZANER: It depends on what age we are talking about and the degree of hearing impairment. I would like to think about those children who are not speaking at all, or who have just a very few words and who have severe to profound hearing impairments. Looking at that population, it is an irrelevancy to be concerned with speech discrimination. We are so hung up on what we consider to be the adult model, whereby we have to compare the performance on speech discrimination unaided and the patient's performance on speech discrimination with different aids, that we refuse to look at this as an irrelevant task for a child who doesn't have expressive language. We also don't know what degree of receptive linguistics skills this youngster has. Certainly Mark Ross' test is great for children for whom it is applicable. With a 2-year old or an 18-month-old child who has not given evidence of receptive language ability, or who has not had the benefit of amplification, forget all that. Get an audiogram that is considered valid.

Find out other audiological details that you feel confident about, such as tolerance problems, acoustic reflexes, or whatever information of that nature is available and do the best job you can to match electroacoustically the needs of the youngster. Then put the hearing aid on and start working.

DR. RUBIN: At this time, there are no clinical speech tests which are not computerized that can be used with the pre-verbal child.

At Lexington, we use aided pure tones and vowels such as /e/, /i/, /a/, and /ou/, a response to name, and simple language. That is about the limit of what can be done clinically with a 6-month-old baby. If the child is sitting unsupported, he will localize to warbled pure tones and to speech. Meanwhile, the mother and child are followed in our educational setting where we can observe them. Only then can we begin to have an understanding of how the child is responding in his acoustic environment with and without amplification. It cannot be accomplished in a sound-proofed chamber in one or two test sessions.

MRS. GRAMMATICO: I don't think it is possible for any one person managing the hearing impaired to collect empirical evidence saying exactly what aid should be prescribed for a very young child independently. This has to be a team approach. The way in which we do this is to help, or assist, the audiologist in an educational setting. The child is first given a clinical evaluation, using as many things as is appropriate for his age level and language development. This clinical information is forwarded to us at the school where we use a master hearing aid with various slopes of amplification curves. We plot, on an educational form, the strategy used (the teaching-learning strategy that is used during each session) and the child's response to this. When we have collected this information on a daily basis from 4 to 6 weeks, depending on the age and the responsiveness of the child, a summary of our information is sent to the audiologist. Those audiologists who work very closely with us are at the San Francisco Hearing and Speech Center. We now have a second affiliated program there that came into being 2 years ago. It has two self-contained classes with children and the audiologists at Franklin Hospital. We have found this to be a good way, probably not the best way, but a good way, in which to collect information that is valuable for these children. I believe that we cannot hold back the educational process for any period of time. What I am suggesting is that these ongoing evaluations that are done functionally in the school setting use cognitively based material as the content for the development of listening skills. The child simply gets a lesson every single day from the cognitive content to develop the listening skills. The inevitable outgrowth is language and speech.

STAPEDIUS MUSCLE REFLEX AND TOLERANCE LEVELS

ANDY BRANDON (AUDIENCE MEMBER): How do you use stapedial reflexes to determine tolerance during the fitting of hearing aids?

DR. McCANDLESS: There is some controversy as to the role or the relationship of the stapedial reflex to overload. The reflex corresponds almost precisely to the point where significant temporary threshold shift occurs, suggesting a physiological and psychoacoustic form of overload. Therefore, if the acoustic reflex is present and carefully measured, it can serve as a basic reference for overload. This doesn't mean that, if it triggers, it is too much. It means that, if the acoustic reflex with a hearing aid goes into a state of rather constant contraction, it is too much. In other words, since speech is an interrupted, highly variable signal, people will tolerate occasional contractions of muscle. We do it all the time when we talk. When the muscle goes into a rather constant state of tonic contraction, then people do not like this over a period of time. This is why we can tolerate rock music. There are periods of relaxation.

The correlation between stapedial muscle reflex and the threshold of discomfort can be used as a general estimate of maximum power output. It is very helpful. The problem is that, as hearing loss becomes greater, the incidence of the presence of the reflex disappears. Above 70 dB, the reflexes occur in only about 50 or 60% of the cases. At that point, it is not valuable at all. It is helpful, then, for those who have less loss. The interesting thing is that, when the reflex is absent, the threshold of discomfort will go up linearly. Again, empirical data may be used. This is what we do now with charts and simply interpolate where it might be, or the measure itself can be taken. Both procedures are helpful. We've been able to try this on children below age 1 year with 40-dB losses. It is particularly helpful in the mild and moderate loss cases. Run it out on a chart recorder, put the impedance probe in the other ear, and turn the gain up and down. It is a fascinating thing to watch with a controlled input.

EFFECT OF DRUGS ON THE ACOUSTIC REFLEX

DR. RUBIN: We have several children here at Lexington who are on long range medication like phenobarbital. During impedance testing, phenobarbital seems to eliminate the stapedius muscle reflex. What happens in daily situations to these children?

DR. McCANDLESS: There is some controversy as to the effect of these drugs on the muscle itself. For example, some people think there is a latency shift. Some people think there is an amplitude shift. Some people think it knocks it right out. With phenobarbital, I don't think there would be a drastic change, but there are some drugs which do change the level on the order of 4 or 5 dB. This is an area we don't know too much about. The question is, "Are sounds more comfortable to these kids, or are they less comfortable, because it's inoperative?" I can't answer that. It's a new area and we've got more to learn.

STIMULI ELICITING THE ACOUSTIC REFLEX

DR. GARDINER (AUDIENCE MEMBER): What input signal is used in testing for the stapedial reflex with hearing aids?

DR. McCANDLESS: We tried broad band noise, narrow band noise, pure tones, speech, and environmental noise. A narrow band noise takes more energy to elicit the reflex. We still feel that speech is probably the best measure. It is somewhat variant, but a good speech sample can be found which does not have a lot of peaks. We find that this corresponds very, very closely with what we like to have in maximum power outputs. Speech spectrum noise is fine because it corresponds almost precisely.

DR. WHITE: In regard to input signals, someone in our group is looking into the possibility of using multiple voices or speech babble as an eliciting signal. Their argument is that the spectrum has more interesting temporal characteristics than filtered noise.

DR. RUBIN: How many voices do you use for speech babble?

DR. WHITE: Several tapes were prepared going from what sounds like minimum to us, which is about six up to 12 or 15 voices, and we're going to see if that matters. It sounds as if above eight there is not much difference.

DR. GERSTMAN: What is good babble? We have a good babble on our tape. We took three women and three men and we had them read "cold" running speech and then listened to the six of them talking and we still heard words. That bothered us because we wanted it to be a background. We randomized a second set of tapes of the same material and threw them in behind the first six, and then we had 12 speakers. When they are babbling you can't recognize any words.

VIBROTACTILE RESPONSES IN CHILDREN

AUDIENCE MEMBER: Is it my understanding that you are working with children with an absence of a cochlea? Would you mind tracing the pathway of sound and what the result is to the central nervous system?

DR. ROSS: These cases wouldn't be getting any sound, but they would be getting vibrotactile responses presumably.

DR. GERSTMAN: We are just assuming they would not get any sound.

MALE VERSUS FEMALE SPEECH SIGNALS

AUDIENCE MEMBER: In doing evaluations with some patients I found that my voice as a woman results in poorer discrimination scores than some of the taped discrimination tests where there is a male voice. Is there a taped discrimination test with a woman's voice?

DR. ROSS: Don Harris did a tape years ago which was a combination speech study where he used a male, female, and child eating a submarine sandwich.

DR. CAUSEY: The Los Angeles Otological Group has a tape with a male voice as well as a female voice. If you will write to them, they will send you back a price list.

DR. ROSS: The modified rhyme test has three different speakers and is commercially available. This is an interesting point because several studies have shown talker-intelligibility interactions and differences.

DR. HARDICK: Pitch of the voice may well be a variable of some importance to hearing-impaired people. Hearing-impaired people can divide the world into good speakers and bad speakers, and it is surprising how many of each sex there are in those groups. It is rather nondiscriminatory. About a year ago, I had some students stand with their backs to the class. They gave a discrimination test in a background of speech babble. This was a tape that was made 10 years ago on which there were 30 speakers. The level of the noise was adjusted so that all our normal hearing college students would get 100% of the items correct. By the same token, no one hit bottom. Each student took a turn in front of the classroom, and then we scored the test results and ranked the students in terms of speaker intelligibility. One of the females turned out to be the most intelligible. If I had to guess in the beginning that she would turn out to be the most intelligible, I probably would not have guessed it. One of the males was at the bottom of the heap. One of the students, who was a hearing aid dealer working on his master's degree, then taped the most intelligible speaker, the least intelligible speaker, and one in the middle, and presented the tape to 24 hearing-impaired people. He asked these individuals to rank order these speakers on the basis of intelligibility. In addition to that, he had them take the test and they confirmed the rank order. Two of these speakers ended up being females—the one at the bottom was a male. That tape was played to a broad spectrum kind of hearing loss, but there was almost unanimous agreement. The point of this is that male versus female voice is certainly a variable, and we have not given the attention to it that we should have, either in the development of tapes, the choice of speakers, or the range of speakers.

DR. HARRIS: In our laboratory, Miss Barbara Kirk did a study like that. There were numbers of men and numbers of women speakers—five of each—and they were ranked by intelligibility tests. Out of the top five, there were about three women. Our conclusion was that the U. S. Navy ought to have women telephone talkers throughout the service.

RICHARD STEPKIN (AUDIENCE MEMBER): Do you think that studying the acoustic reflex may reduce potential noise-induced hearing loss with hearing aids?

AIDED THRESHOLD SHIFT AND THE ACOUSTIC REFLEX

DR. McCANDLESS: The acoustic reflex on normal subjects occurs at 90 to 95 dB. There is quite a range. If the signal is loud enough for the reflex to stay in a reasonable contracted state, the noise risk criterion goes up. In other words, this corresponds to a long-term exposure criteria. It may be accidental, but it does correspond quite nicely. Any time a sound pressure of about 90 to 100 dB is reached, there is a danger area for people with mild or normal hearing losses. Just because the reflex contracts, it doesn't mean it's all right. It still can be hazardous.

What has happened in this whole question of the possible damage caused by hearing aids is that people fortunately adjust the volume since they can't adjust the maximum power output. They adjust the volume so that the input signal plus the gain is just below this level. A child couldn't adjust the volume, and that's where the danger occurs. Adults do not have damage because they *do* adjust the volume control down just below this level. Infants are another story. Someone gave the example of the fussy infant this morning. How do you know how much amplification to give a baby? We see our auropalpebral reflexes in older children with amplification and change not the gain but the maximum power output until that disappears and everything smoothes out. There is no reason to think that the ears of children act any differently than infants. They behave precisely the same way.

DR. MADELL: We fit a child with an aid for a period of time and then measure the child's thresholds immediately before putting the hearing aid on. We are measuring the child's temporary threshold shift to find the most suitable maximum power output for that child.

DR. ZANER: In fitting aids with young children, we tend to equate overloading with maximum power output, whereas my concern is in the gain. It is easier to figure out how little gain you should provide in order to just reach threshold and not to overload.

DR. WILBER: My concern is that the government has said that adults should not be at noise levels exceeding 90 dB A for an 8-hour day; that it is dangerous to do so. That means, perhaps, that people should not wear hearing aids with a gain of more than 30 dB because that would put them in the situation of 90 dB A if anybody is talking.

NOISE-INDUCED THRESHOLD SHIFT IN THE PATHOLOGICAL EAR

DR. ROSS: Doesn't the actual shift relate to the preexisting loss? If a normal hearing person spends an 8-hour day at 90 dB A, he will have a certain amount of shift. If he has a 70-dB loss and is exposed to 90 dB A, the amount of the shift would be less.

DR. WILBER: It makes absolutely no difference because the 90 dB A is getting to the same cochlea unless that 70-dB loss is conductive.

DR. ROSS: No. The actual amount of permanent threshold shift is less when there is a preexisting loss because generally the same structure is being damaged.

DR. WILBER: We are not really sure about it because it depends on where the damage is in the cochlea and what other kinds of damage are being created.

THE UTOPIAN HEARING AID

DR. HARRIS: We have a paper by Hyman Goldberg, the very knowledgeable president of Dyna-aura Laboratories, entitled, "The Utopian Hearing Aid." He described an aid which the subject cannot adjust but which is preadjusted for him. How close are we to such an aid?

DR. SINCLAIR: Hyman designed that aid and, if you will listen to him, he will tell you he has got it. His aid fits particular losses. It is not a universal utopian, but utopian for particular losses. Industry does not have a utopian aid, but there is a lot of work going on. We are concerned in the industry, at the moment, in just producing the aids we do produce. Features such as directional, electret mikes, better compression, attack, and recovery times are very basic developments. We are fitting a wider range of losses rather than coming to a utopian aid. There are more aids, and not all these features are found in each aid. The directional characteristic is not found in every aid and it is not good for every loss. We are trying to add features to existing aids.

DR. HARRIS: You are too close to the problem, Dr. Sinclair. I look into developments about every 3 to 5 years and, every time I look, a revolution has transpired in the hearing aid technical industry.

DR. SINCLAIR: Yes, but unfortunately these revolutions are slow. For example, Don Causey was having great success with CROS fittings. He presented a 30% statistic, but the industry fitting of CROS is far below that. It is an interesting statistic that his fitting is 30% and the industry fitting is perhaps 5%. They are quite far apart. When these new developments come out, they are tried on and perhaps overfit. I agree that we tend to think that each aid is going to be the utopian aid and solve our problems, but I have yet to see that aid. It just doesn't work that way. I don't see any utopian aid yet. Individual designers have got their own utopian aid. I've got an aid I like, too. I'll call it utopian, but it really isn't.

SPECIAL AIDS DESIGNED FOR CHILDREN

DR. RUBIN: Do you have any aids on the market especially designed for children?

DR. SINCLAIR: When I talk to audiologists and they start talking about standards, they try to use the standard to sometimes tell industry what to design. One of the things audiologists are trying to design is a children's aid. Manufacturers have not been very successful with it in general. I don't quite understand why. I do know that several of the firms are now working, mainly under pressure from audiologists, clinics, and the schools, to come up with more rugged hearing aids for children. Aids today are not children's aids. The most destructive person to an aid is still the child. We built a hearing aid for one of the Bears football players who has a hearing problem. It was required that it be in a helmet and that he could throw his helmet off. He throws it on the ground when he gets a touchdown or something. We built this aid in the helmet on a flexible circuit and had the earphone dangling because he had to be able to rip it off. Every time the Bears played a game, I expected to get a telephone call the next day saying that we had better fix that aid. That aid went through the whole season without a fault. Yet, if I built an aid and gave it to a child, the next day it would be back with the child having found a way to break it. We don't have a good solution for the child. There are various companies working on it. Again I'll say, *"We do not have a good child's aid in the industry."* Give a child any aid and they'll find a way of damaging it. We do need some design input and would welcome ideas.

ELECTROACOUSTICAL SYSTEMS FOR CHILDREN

DR. RUBIN: Audiologists are not talking about a robust aid necessarily, but an aid with flexible acoustical characteristics, designed for children's use. Have you given that any consideration?

DR. SINCLAIR: I have not had any pressure put on me to design aids which are different for children from aids for adults, except for a school population with only a corner audiogram. There would be a special aid for that population. As far as the normal losses, I don't know of any difference in approach acoustically. Designers found that getting the body aid off the children is the problem, especially for teenagers, and there are a lot of requests for a hearing aid to replace body aids.

EXTERNAL RECEIVERS ON EAR LEVEL AIDS

DR. SINCLAIR: One of the problems is that if you use the internal receivers that are inside the behind-the-ear aid, you get different acoustics than you do if you use that external receiver. It is not possible technically to duplicate a button receiver with a small internal receiver, and that becomes a problem. If children have been using a body aid and button phones, they will find a difference when fitted with an internal receiver. There are aids on the market which are behind the ear with external receivers for that reason. It is a very small market, and very few aids are made. Our company made only 100 of them because we didn't think we would hit a big market and we sold thousands of them.

There are also certain behind-the-ear units with mike-tel switches and tel coils in them, but perhaps not of the strength required.

DR. RUBIN: Yes, that's correct. The mike-tel switch in an ear-level aid also only allows the child to receive a signal. The child cannot monitor his own speech. We would like an ear-level aid with the same capability as a body aid which has a "both" position; then the child could use the aid in a looped classroom.

DR. SINCLAIR: I wish it weren't so, but it is a small market, and we are already in a small market. That's one of the problems. Over a period of time, with enough input from people, such as questions like your own, manufacturers will respond. Don Causey knows this with the Veterans Administration. He has received a high frequency aid, for example. Just keep asking for it and it will happen, but it might seem awfully slow.

DR. ZANER: With regard to the external button on the ear-level aid, Dr. Sinclair said that those aids are provided in order to bridge the gap between a child using a body aid and a behind-the-ear aid. Do you think that the child could eventually get used to the behind-the-ear aid and then not need the other, or is it really better to have that outside receiver and, if so, why don't we just do that?

DR. SINCLAIR: I'm not sure. The request came because there were children going into their teens who refused to wear the body aid. When we put conventional behind-the-ear units on them, they would sometimes pretend it worked. However, they weren't doing as well. They threw away something by going from their body aid to that behind-the-ear unit, but they would not wear the body aid. We traced it to this receiver, which was one of the variables, and we were able to build the external receiver. We asked kids to wear it and try it, and it did come closer to the performance of the body aid. Again, it is not utopian, but it was a try to bridge a problem, and the substitution of a button receiver for an internal receiver was one of the tricks that did it.

DR. ROSS: What precisely did you find with the ear-level aid with an internal receiver that didn't make it as satisfactory as a body aid? There are many ear-level aids on the market that appear to have the same response as body aids.

DR. SINCLAIR: There are two differences. One of the differences not seen very often is the way ear-level aids go into saturation. They go into saturation quite differently, and the maximum for the different frequencies is quite different for a button phone and internal phone. A 90-dB sound pressure curve will reveal the difference. It is both saturation and the frequency response.

DR. McCANDLESS: Is there a difference in the frequency response above 3,000 Hz? Some of the high frequency aids with an internal receiver extend out, to 3,800, but they are down 10 dB or so at the maximum power output. In other words, although the frequency response extends, the maximum power output for some of the receivers is 10 or 15 dB below what it is on the conventional body aids. Perhaps this extended half-octave makes a difference.

NEED FOR QUALITY EDUCATION
FOR HEARING-IMPAIRED CHILDREN

MRS. GRAMMATICO: I'm not an audiologist, and I believe that a child can have the best amplifier system in the world most appropriately selected, but, without quality education intervention, the child will not develop his potential. Certainly adults have reached formal operational reasoning and can take and process small pieces of information. Children, on the other hand, from 0 to 2 years, are in a sensorimotor stage of development, and then go into preoperational, concrete operations. Is audiology taking a look at this?

DR. McCANDLESS: That is a very accurate observation. It is very difficult to couple what we know about the ear in isolation to its complex functioning, and then to try to make accurate predictions on the basis of fittings about what is going to happen educationally. Obviously, we can't. We can have educational success with poor hearing aid fittings and vice versa. We can have the best hearing aid in the world and poor educational success. Obviously, it is a combination that we would like to achieve. We know some of the things that make educational successes. We know fewer things which make good hearing aid fittings, and the question is, "How can we, without using adult criteria, make a reasonable guess as to what is the best for the time?"

We cannot make the same distinctions, even as far as severity, with young children, as we can with adults. There have to be some dichotomies that children have a hearing loss or they don't, or they have a mild or moderate hearing loss. Because we know very little about configuration and dynamics, we are left with the severity and the slope. We make some estimate about site of lesion and cause and then take the inferential data that we have on older children and adults and transmit this down to children with the assumption that the pathological ear doesn't work all that differently in infants. It doesn't change from 1 month to 4 years. Why should we treat these children any differently than an adult? Why don't we limit children as we do adults, instead of putting big powerful aids on them? We are not utilizing the information that we have.

DR. CAUSEY: I don't know what a hearing aid for children would consist of to make it any different from a hearing aid for an adult, unless its rugged performance would be considered. We give adults tests in the clinic with four different hearing aids, all judged to be the finest quality, and four different models. Then we send them home with each one for a 2-week period and then bring them back. At the end of those trial periods, there is not going to be any difference in performance among those four hearing aids. In other words, there is going to be a period of learning that takes place, and the person's performance with that hearing aid at the end of the 2-week period is not going to be different from one aid to another. In fact, you can send an individual home with a poor hearing aid and, given a long enough time, his performance will equal that with a good hearing aid.

The point with young children is to be careful as to the type of hearing aid you provide. Make sure it is of the finest quality, see that it gets to the child as soon as possible and that you do not provide more gain than the child needs. There will never be a hearing aid for a child different than that for an adult except with regard to the ruggedness of the construction.

DR. ZANER: I agree with Mrs. Grammatico that the child will not achieve unless there is excellent intervention after amplification. The opposite of that is also true. Namely, relatively poor amplification or reasonably good amplification with good intervention will also produce good results.

The important point to be aware of is the developmental sequence in children. A child cannot be expected to participate in a test that is created for an adult. My concern today is to note that, even where children do have words with which to test, the linguistic system of that child is a very different linguistic system from the adventitiously deafened or hearing-impaired adult who can use auditory memory. Looking for responses to animal noises, responses to doorbells and airplanes, and so on, is in no way a substitute for the discrimination tests that we give adults with speech.

GOOD AMPLIFICATION VERSUS POOR AMPLIFICATION

DR. DOERFLER (AUDIENCE MEMBER): There is no doubt in my mind that there is a world of difference between an amplification system that has good characteristics in delivering speech signals to an impaired ear and one that has high distortion or other inadequacies. If one's background is an educational one, one recognizes that quality educational intervention is critical. That's certainly true, but the enabling device very often is the amplifier. What can be accomplished by educational intervention is going to be severely limited with an inadequate type of delivery system of sound.

NEED FOR TEACHER-AUDIOLOGIST COOPERATION

DR. ROSS: As a final comment, we have been separating the diagnostic audiological from the educational, and we are finding some of our results inadequate because the audiologists have not been in both areas. The action is in an educational setting. Those programs that we hear the best things about have the audiologists and the teachers working together. The diagnostic and the educational functions are working hand in hand. Then we are able, as audiologists, to do the best we can while teachers get the best from the children with good amplification.

FUTURE
PERSPECTIVES

FUTURE DEVELOPMENTS IN HEARING AIDS

Leo G. Doerfler

The task of peering into a clouded, yet tantalizing, future regarding hearing aids and their optimal use calls for a recognition of several facts, as well as a willingness to sift among numerous signs and select those which may turn out to be significant portents. The "Proceedings of the Lexington Hearing Aid Conference" was one of those all-too-rare opportunities for scientists, engineers, educators, and clinicians to report experiences, react to theories, and to interact in a hopefully productive manner. The future will tell whether positive changes in hearing aids and their usage will result.

The most significant fact to be recognized appears to be that hearing aid electrotechnology has progressed to the point where engineers possess the capability of producing, almost on demand, wearable devices which can manipulate the parameters of amplification in ways undreamt of perhaps a decade or two ago. And, in recognition of consumer attitudes, these devices can be packaged in a cosmetically acceptable manner.

The question that the hearing aid engineers face is a simple one which apparently is yet to be answered: which parameters are significant, and how are they to be altered? Part of the answer appears reasonably clear; we will require, well into the future, an array of instruments and/or controls which will provide the professional with the armamentarium required for meeting the complex auditory needs of the user,

Even this partial answer begs the fundamental question: what are these needs and how are they to be specified? The answer appears to lie in the direction of the development of what some have called "a psychophysics of impaired hearing." But the solution will undoubtedly turn out to be more complex than this; there are many variations of impaired hearing, and when these are even partially specified, we still will be faced with many nagging practical questions.

Will manufacturers find it economically feasible to turn out relatively small numbers of numerous models of hearing aids to meet the particular amplification needs of these small populations? Or, if it is feasible to build into a single hearing aid or several aids all of the desirable parameters, would this step be counterproductive to our goal of generally reducing the unit cost of manufacturing hearing aids?

The highly competitive nature of the hearing aid manufacturing business, plus the history of its responsiveness to demonstrated need of specific populations, such as prelingually hearing-impaired children, suggests that we will see in the future an increasing variety of hearing aids designed to produce the desired manipulations of auditory signals. Thus, we will have the tools with which to do a better job, but at an increasing economic cost.

PRESCRIPTION FITTING

The term "prescription fitting" engenders mixed reactions among professionals because of its medical implications. However, there are strong indications of a trend in this direction for several reasons. First is the increased use of specific audiological information gathered through both standard procedures and newer tests, including tympanometry, auditory reflex measures, speech and noise interference tests, etc., which help in specifying the required amplification parameters.

Second is the remarkable growth in successful usage of what I prefer to call "in-the-earmold" rather than "in-the-ear hearing aids." Manufacturers appear to be increasingly adept in manipulating the electronic parameters of these aids in accordance with specified needs, and still apparently remain within reasonable quality control limits. There is a good probability that, within the next few years, a majority of hearing aids will be of this type as the feedback problem is solved.

Third, the number of audiologists and audiology centers becoming directly involved in the dispensing of hearing aids will increase gradually in the next few years, and the direct specification of amplification parameters, along with the increased potential for continuing monitoring of patients resulting from dispensing, will prove to be a factor in encouraging "prescription." There will be some increase in the use of a "master hearing aid" for fitting purposes, but the majority of audiologists will continue to utilize a combination of test results, clinical experience and a small degree of clinical "hunch."

DISTRIBUTION SYSTEMS

The present decade has seen the evolutionary beginnings of a substantive alteration in the manner in which hearing aids are delivered into the hands (and, hopefully, ears) of the consumer. For over 40 years, aids have been dispensed directly by dealers, generally as a direct purchase by the consumer, sometimes on the recommendation of a professional. Although some users have been helped by this system, apparently a significant number have not been well served, judging by the results of independent surveys and the recurring reports of dissatisfied users and nonusers.

Increasing consumer pressure, growing professional interest in improving services, and governmental concern in the areas of quality of service and economics have conspired to place the commercial dealer in a difficult position. As a legitimate businessman selling a prosthetic device, he now finds himself accused of not performing as a professional, a role which he never claimed. His immediate reaction has been to obtain professional training, a task which, with few exceptions, he cannot carry out in the absence of long-term training.

Nevertheless, attempts are being made by some manufacturers, trade associations, and a few community colleges to recoup the traditional hearing dealer role in this manner. Although some consumers will be aided by those dealers who strive to improve their limited information of what is essentially professional audiological and otological knowledge, it appears that these attempts to shore up an inadequate system will not be fruitful in the long run. One is reminded of such analogies as early communication by means of the pony express. The answer to improvement in communication could not be achieved by improvements in horse breeding, more comfortable saddles, or stronger riders, but had to come through the development of a new system. And thus it appears to be developing with the system of rehabilitating the hearing impaired through amplification.

Clearly, there will continue to be an intermix of commercial hearing aid dealers along with a growing number of professional dispensers for the foreseeable future, especially in less populated areas of the country. And, of course, some small portion of the present dealer population will obtain professional training to equip themselves for the future. But pressures from consumers and third-party payers for comprehensive professional services, along with a growing commitment on the part of audiologists toward improved rehabilitation, will play a major role in this evolutionary step.

For some persons, especially those involved in academic audiology, the prospect of audiologists dispensing hearing aids in a unified hearing health care delivery system raises the question of a possible conflict of interest since the sale of a prosthetic device is involved. This point of view ignores the fact that a potential conflict of interest exists in any situation where the individual making a judgment or recommendation stands to benefit from the subsequent action taken by the recipient of his advice, regardless of whether or not a tangible purchase is made. Thus, a public school speech therapist has an inherent conflict of interest when he or she diagnoses an articulation problem in a child and places the child on his or her therapy program, for the therapist's job is dependent upon having an appropriate caseload. A physician has his or her income directly affected by the nature of any medical recommendations made. Even the academic budget of a graduate training program may be dependent upon the size of its student therapy load, which of course is dependent, in turn, upon the diagnostic decisions made by faculty and supervisors. So it is clearly naive to develop a unique response to the question of possible conflict of interest in the case of an audiologist because a prosthetic device is involved.

How then do we achieve this trust in professional areas when there is this implicit conflict of interest? Primarily through a cultural ethic which is brought about by years of professional training, proper models of behaviors, and a code of ethics which deals not with economics and fiscal controls but with legitimate professional concerns such as a monitoring of the professional appropriate areas. The profession of audiology appears to have matured to the point where it has developed this cultural and professional ethic and can escape the narrow bureaucratic impulse to control our behavior through ill-advised economic strictures. We must be concerned with the quality of care and monitor this through peer group evaluation, while the economics involved are handled by individual patient choice and third-party payers: in essence, the marketplace.

THE HARD OF HEARING AND HEARING AID USAGE

While the number of hearing-impaired persons has apparently continued to increase along with the increase in the general population, the number of hearing aids dispensed has not reflected this increase. Industry figures indicate that sales of hearing aids for the past 5 years have remained in the 600,000- to 640,000-unit range, with little or no increase during the current year, a figure which is perhaps 5 to 10% of the hearing-impaired population which might benefit from the use of a hearing aid. The reasons usually given for this disappointing record include increased surgical restoration of hearing and the current economic situation.

The above figures are interesting in a number of ways. Manufacturers and commercial dealers generally indicate that a majority of hearing aid sales at the dealer level are repeat sales, suggesting that the current dispensing model is not successful in drawing new hearing aid users into the system, at least to a desirable degree. In contrast, several of the newer dispensing models, either audiology center, audiologist-otologist, or private practice audiologist dispensing, report that a majority of their dispensing involves new, rather than repeat, hearing aid users. One such center at the Eye and Ear Hospital of Pittsburgh has found that approximately 90% of the first 1,000 hearing aids dispensed were with first time hearing aid users. In time, of course, this percentage will decrease, but the strong implication is that these newer models of dispensing will serve the desired function of increasing the number of persons using hearing aids successfully.

INNOVATIVE HEARING RESTORATION TECHNIQUES

Over the years a number of physiologists, surgeons, and experimental audiologists have speculated about the possibility of some form of direct electrical stimulation of some portion of the auditory system, thus bypassing a damaged or nonfunctioning structure. These speculations have ranged from direct stimulation of the cochlea, the eighth nerve, or even the auditory cortex. The deterrent, apart from the surgical difficulties, has been that the function of the bypassed structure in the transmission or encoding of the signal or impulse-system would have to be replaced by some electronic substitute, and/or the individual would have to be retrained to interpret a substantially altered set of sensations.

The latest foray into this area has been the surgical implantation of an electrode into essentially the first turn of the scala tympani, which, with associated external electronics, produces electrical stimulation of a portion of the cochlea directly. Several dozen persons have volunteered for this surgery; it has been carried out at three locations in this country and is being considered abroad. In addition, an independent evaluation of the audiological, psychoacoustic, vestibular, and psychological aspects of this procedure on a number of persons is being pursued.

At this point in time, it appears that the major result has been a restoration of a sensation of sound to those undergoing the procedure. This sound sensation enables the individual to regain the sense of awareness of a sound-filled world and to make some simple gross discriminations. Restoration of hearing, in the sense of understanding speech without visual clues, does not appear to have been achieved.

The major positive aspect of this development has been to focus attention upon an area of clinical research which will serve as a magnet for basic researchers from a number of traditional disciplines. Funds will be attracted, and questions will be raised which can and will be answered. Selection of patients will have to be dealt with, various electrode arrays tried out, improved electronics provided, and attention be paid to retraining of patients to interpret and benefit from the altered sensation which is being delivered to the brain. Although some researchers might feel uncomfortable in that the traditional gradual scientific path of extensive animal and laboratory research has not preceded the actual clinical experimental trials in this instance, and some scientists decry the manner in which the public relations aspects of the matter have been handled, bold steps, such as these, appear to serve as catalysts which force the scientific and clinical community to focus upon a process, and this can have far-reaching positive results.

APPENDIX A

LEGISLATION AFFECTING THE IMPLEMENTATION OF HEARING AID STANDARDS

94th CONGRESS
1st Session
H. R. 11124

IN THE HOUSE OF REPRESENTATIVES

December 11, 1975

Mr. Rogers (for himself, Mr. Satterfield, Mr. Preyer, Mr. Symington, Mr. Scheuer, Mr. Waxman, Mr. Hefner, Mr. Florio, Mr. Carney, Mr. Maguire, Mr. Carter, Mr. Broyhill, Mr. Hastings, and Mr. Heinz) introduced the following bill; which was referred to the Committee on Interstate and Foreign Commerce

A BILL

To amend the Federal Food, Drug, and Cosmetic Act to provide for the safety and effectiveness of medical devices intended for human use, and for other purposes.

Be it enacted by the Senate and House of Representatives of the United States of America in Congress assembled,

SHORT TITLE AND TABLE OF CONTENTS

Section 1. (a) This Act may be cited as the "Medical Device Amendments of 1975".

(b) Whenever in this Act an amendment is expressed in terms of an amendment to a section or other provision, the reference shall be considered to be made to a section or other provision of the Federal Food, Drug, and Cosmetic Act.

231

TABLE OF CONTENTS

Sec. 2. Regulation of medical devices–*continued*
> "(e) Restricted devices.
> "(f) Good manufacturing practice requirements.
> "(g) Exemption for devices for investigational use.
> "(h) Release of safety and effectiveness information.
> "(i) Proceedings of advisory panels and committees.
> "(j) Traceability requirements.
> "(k) Research and development.
> "(l) Transitional provisions for devices considered as new drugs or antibiotic drugs.

"Sec. 521. State and local requirements respecting devices.
> "(a) General rule.
> "(b) Exempt requirements."

Sec. 3. Conforming amendments.
> (a) Amendments to section 201.
> (b) Amendments to section 301.
> (c) Amendments to section 304.
> (d) Amendments to section 501.
> (e) Amendments to section 502.
> (f) Amendments to section 801.

Sec. 4. Registration of device manufacturers.
Sec. 5. Device established and official names.
Sec. 6. Inspections relating to devices.
Sec. 7. Administrative restraint.
Sec. 8. Confidential information; presumption.
Sec. 9. Color additives.
Sec. 10. Assistance for small manufacturers of devices.

REGULATION OF MEDICAL DEVICES

Sec. 2. Chapter V is amended by adding after section 512 the following new sections:

"CLASSIFICATION OF DEVICES INTENDED FOR HUMAN USE
"Device Classes

"Sec. 513. (a) (1) There are established the following classes of devices intended for human use:

"(A) Class I, General Controls.—

"(i) A device for which the controls authorized by or under section 501, 502, 510, 516, 518, 519, or 520 or any combination of such sections are sufficient to provide reasonable assurance of the safety and effectiveness of the device.

"(ii) A device for which insufficient information exists to determine that the controls referred to in clause (i) are sufficient to provide reasonable assurance of the safety and effectiveness of the device or to establish a performance standard to provide such assurance, but because it—

"(I) is not purported or represented to be for a use which is of substantial importance in supporting, sustaining, or preventing impairment of human life or health, and

"(II) does not present a potential unreasonable risk of illness or injury,

is to be regulated by the controls referred to in clause (i).

"(B) Class II, Performance Standards.—A device which cannot be classified as a class I device because the controls authorized by or under sections 501, 502, 510, 516, 518, 519, and 520 by themselves are insufficient to provide reasonable assurance of the safety and effectiveness of the device, for which there is sufficient information to establish a performance standard to provide such assurance, and for which it is therefore necessary to establish for the device a performance standard under section 514 to provide reasonable assurance of its safety and effectiveness.

"(C) Class III, Premarket Approval.—A device which because—

"(i) it (I) cannot be classified as a class I device because insufficient information exists to determine that the controls authorized by or under sections 501, 502, 510, 516, 518, 519, and 520 are sufficient to provide reasonable assurance of the safety and effectiveness of the device and (II) cannot be classified as a class II device because insufficient information exists for the establishment of a performance standard to provide reasonable assurance of its safety and effectiveness, and

"(ii) (I) is purported or represented to be for a use which is of substantial importance in supporting, sustaining, or preventing impairment of human life or health, or

"(II) presents a potential unreasonable risk of illness or injury,
is to be subject, in accordance with section 515, to premarket approval to provide reasonable assurance of its safety and effectiveness.

If there is not sufficient information to establish a performance standard for a device to provide reasonable assurance of its safety and effectiveness, the Secretary may conduct such activities as may be necessary to develop or obtain such information.

"(2) For purposes of this section and sections 514 and 515, the safety and effectiveness of a device are to be determined—

"(A) with respect to the persons for whose use the device is represented or intended,

"(B) with respect to the conditions of use prescribed, recommended, or suggested in the labeling of the device, and

"(C) weighing any probable benefit to health from the use of the device against any probable risk of injury or illness from such use.

"(3) (A) Except as authorized by subparagraph (B), the effectiveness of a device is, for purposes of this section and sections 514 and 515, to be determined, in accordance with regulations promulgated by the Secretary, on the basis of well-controlled investigations, including clinical investigations where appropriate, by experts qualified by training and experience to evaluate the effectiveness of the device, from which investigations it can fairly and responsibly be concluded by qualified experts that the device will have the effect it purports or is represented to have under the conditions of use prescribed, recommended, or suggested in the labeling of the device.

"(B) If the Secretary determines that there exists valid scientific evidence (other than evidence derived from investigations described in subparagraph (A))—

"(i) which is sufficient to determine the effectiveness of a device, and

"(ii) from which it can fairly and responsibly be concluded by qualified experts that the device will have the effect it purports or is represented to have under the conditions of use prescribed, recommended, or suggested in the labeling of the device,

then, for purposes of this section and sectons 514 and 515, the Secretary may authorize the effectiveness of the device to be determined on the basis of such evidence.

"Classification; Classification Panels

"(b) (1) For purposes of—

"(A) determining which devices intended for human use should be subject to the requirements of general controls, performance standards, or premarket approval, and

"(B) providing notice to the manufacturers and importers of such devices to enable them to prepare for the application of such requirements to devices manufactured or imported by them,

the Secretary shall classify all such devices into the classes established by subsection (a). For the purpose of securing recommendations with respect to the classification of devices, the Secretary shall establish panels of experts or use panels of experts established before the date of the enactment of this section, or both. Section 14 of the Federal Advisory Committee Act shall not apply to the duration of a panel established under this paragraph.

"(2) The Secretary shall appoint to each panel established under paragraph (1) persons who are qualified by training and experience to evaluate the safety and effectiveness of the devices to be referred to the panel and who, to the extent feasible, possess skill in the use of, or experience in the development, manufacture, or utilization of, such devices. The Secretary shall make appointments to each panel so that each panel shall consist of members with adequately diversified expertise in such fields as clinical and administrative medicine, engineering, biological and physical sciences, and other related professions. In addition, each panel shall include as nonvoting members a representative of consumer interests and a representative of interests of the device manufacturing industry. Scientific, trade, and consumer organizations shall be afforded an opportunity to nominate individuals for appointment to the panels. No individual who is in the regular full-time employ of the United States and engaged in the administration of this Act may be a member of any panel. The Secretary shall designate one of the members of each panel to serve as chairman thereof.

"(3) Panel members (other than officers or employees of the United States), while attending meetings or conferences of a panel or otherwise engaged in its business, shall be entitled to receive compensation at rates to be fixed by the Secretary, but not at rates exceeding the daily equivalent of the rate in effect for grade GS-18 of the General Schedule, for each day so engaged, including traveltime; and while so serving away from their homes or regular places of business each member may be allowed travel expenses (including per diem in lieu of subsistence) as authorized by section 5703 (b) of title 5, United States Code, for persons in the Government service employed intermittently.

"(4) The Secretary shall furnish each panel with adequate clerical and other necessary assistance.

"Classification Panel Organization and Operation

"(c) (1) The Secretary shall organize the panels according to the various fields of clinical medicine and fundamental sciences in which devices intended for human use are used. The Secretary shall refer a device to be classified under this section to an appropriate panel established or authorized to be used under subsection (b) for its review and for its recommendation respecting the classification of the device and, to the extent practicable, respecting the assignment of a priority for the application of the requirements of section 514 or 515 to the device if the panel recommends that the device be classified in class II or class III. The Secretary shall by regulation prescribe the procedure to be followed by the panels in making their reviews and recommendations. In making their reviews of devices, the panels, to the maximum extent practicable, shall provide an opportunity for interested persons to submit data and views on the classification of the devices.

"(2) (A) Upon completion of a panel's review of a device referred to it under paragraph (1), the panel shall, subject to subparagraphs (B) and (C), submit to the Secretary its recommendation for the classification of the device. Any such recommendation shall (i) contain (I) a summary of the reasons for the recommendation, (II) a summary of the data upon which the recommendation is based, and (III) an identification of the risks to health (if any) presented by the device with respect to which the recommendation is made, and (ii) to the extent practicable, includes a recommendation for the assignment of a priority for the application of the requirements of section 514 or 515 to a device recommended to be classified in class II or class III.

"(B) A recommendation of a panel for the classification of a device in class I shall include a recommendation as to whether the device should be exempted from the requirements of section 510, 519, or 520 (f).

"(C) In the case of a device which has been referred under paragraph (1) to a panel, and which—

"(i) is intended to be implanted in the human body, and

"(ii) (I) has been introduced or delivered for introduction into interstate commerce for commercial distribution on or before the date of enactment of this section, or

"(II) is within a type of device which was so introduced or delivered on or before such date and is substantially equivalent to another device within that type,

such panel shall recommend to the Secretary that the device be classified in class III unless the panel determines that classification of the device in such class is not necessary to provide reasonable assurance of its safety and effectiveness. If a panel does not recommend that such a device be classified in class III, it shall in its recommendation to the Secretary for the classification of the device set forth the reasons for not recommending classification of the device in such class.

"(3) The panels shall submit to the Secretary within one year of the date funds are first appropriated for the implementation of this section their recommendations respecting all devices of a type introduced or delivered for introduction into interstate commerce for commercial distribution on or before the date of the enactment of this section.

"Classification

"(d) (1) Upon receipt of a recommendation from a panel respecting a device, the Secretary shall publish in the Federal Register the panel's recommendation and a proposed regulation classifying such device and shall provide interested persons an opportunity to submit comments on such recommendation and the proposed regulation. After reviewing such comments, the Secretary shall, subject to paragraph (2), by regulation classify such device.

"(2) (A) A regulation under paragraph (1) classifying a device in class I shall prescribe which, if any, of the requirements of section 510, 519, or 520(f) shall not apply to the device.

"(B) A device described in subsection (c) (2) (C) shall be classified in class III unless the Secretary determines that classification of the device in such class is not necessary to provide reasonable assurance of its safety and effectiveness. A proposed regulation under paragraph (1) classifying such a device in a class other than class III shall be accompanied by a statement of the reasons of the Secretary for not classifying such device in such class.

"(3) In the case of devices classified under this subsection in class II and devices classified under this subsection in class III and described in section 515(b) (1), the Secretary may establish priorities which, in his discretion, shall be used in applying sections 514 and 515, as appropriate, to such devices.

"Classification Changes

"(e) Based on new information respecting a device, the Secretary may, upon his own initiative or upon petition of an interested person, by regulation (1) change such device's classification, and (2) revoke, because of the change in classifcation, any regulation or requirement in effect under section 514 or 515 with respect to such device. In the promulgation of such a regulation respecting a device's classification, the Secretary may secure from the panel to which the device was last referred pursuant to subsection (c) a recommendation respecting the proposed change in the device's classification and shall publish in the Federal Register any recommendation submitted to the Secretary by the panel respecting such change. A regulation under this subsection changing the classification of a device from class III to class II may provide that such classification shall not take effect until the effective date of a performance standard established under section 514 for such device.

"Initial Classification of Certain Devices

"(f) (1) Any device intended for human use which was not introduced or delivered for introduction into interstate commerce for commercial distribution before the date of the enactment of this section is classified in class III unless—

"(A) the device—

"(i) is within a type of device (I) which was introduced or delivered for introduction into interstate commerce for commercial distribution on or before such date or (II) which was not so introduced or delivered on or before such date and has been classified in class I or II, and

"(ii) is substantially equivalent to another device within such type, or

"(B) in the case of a device other than a device which is intended to be implanted in the human body, the Secretary in response to a petition submitted under paragraph (2) has classified such device in class I or II.

A device (other than a device which is intended to be implanted in the human body) classified in class III under this paragraph shall be classified in that class until the effective date of an order of the Secretary under paragraph (2) classifying the device in class I or II. The Secretary may not promulgate a regulation under subsection (e) changing the classification of a device which is intended to be implanted in the human body and which is classified in class III under this paragraph before there is in effect for such device an approval under section 515 of an application for premarket approval.

"(2) The manufacturer or importer of a device classified under paragraph (1) (other than a device which is intended to be implanted in the human body) may petition the Secretary (in such form and manner as he shall prescribe) for the issuance of an order classifying the device in class I or class II. Within thirty days of the filing of such a petition, the Secretary shall notify the petitioner of any deficiencies in the petition which prevent the Secretary from making a decision on the petition. Within one hundred and eighty days after the filing of a petition under this paragraph and after affording the petitioner an opportunity for an informal hearing, the Secretary shall, after consultation with the appropriate panel established or authorized to be used under subsection (b), by order either deny the petition or order the classification, in accordance with the criteria prescribed by subsection (a) (1) (A) or (a) (1) (B), of the device in class I or class II.

"Information

"(g) Within sixty days of the receipt of a written request of any person for information respecting the class in which a device has been classified or the requirements applicable to a device under this Act, the Secretary shall provide such person a written statement of the classification (if any) of such device and the requirements of this Act applicable to the device.

"Definitions

"(h) For purposes of this section and sections 501, 510, 514, 515, 519, and 520—

"(1) a reference to 'general controls' is a reference to the controls authorized by or under sections 501, 502, 510, 516, 518, 519, and 520,

"(2) a reference to 'class I', 'class II', or 'class III' is a reference to a class of medical devices described in subparagraph (A), (B), or (C) of subsection (a) (1), and

"(3) a reference to a 'panel under section 513' is a reference to a panel established or authorized to be used under this section.

"PERFORMANCE STANDARDS

"Provisions of Standards

"Sec. 514. (a) (1) The Secretary may by regulation, promulgated in accordance with this section, establish a performance standard for a class II device. A class III device may also be considered a class II device for purposes of establishing a standard for the device under this section if the device has been reclassified as a class II device under a regulation under section 513(e) but such regulation provides that the reclassification is not to take effect until the effective date of such a standard for the device.

"(2) A performance standard established under this section for a device—

"(A) shall include provisions to provide reasonable assurance of its safe and effective performance;

"(B) shall, where necessary to provide reasonable assurance of its safe and effective performance, include—

"(i) provisions respecting the construction, components, ingredients, and properties of the device and its compatibility with power systems and connections to such systems,

"(ii) provisions for the testing (on a sample basis or, if necessary, on an individual basis) of the device or, if it is determined that no other more practicable means are available to the Secretary to assure the conformity of the device to the standard, provisions for the testing (on a sample basis or, if necessary, on an individual basis) by the Secretary or by another person at the direction of the Secretary,

"(iii) provisions for the measurement of the performance characteristics of the device,

"(iv) provisions requiring that before the device is introduced or delivered for introduction into interstate commerce for commercial distribution the results of each or of certain of the tests of the device required to be made under clause (ii) show that the device is in conformity with the portions of the standard for which the test or tests were required, and

"(v) a provision requiring that the sale and distribution of the device be restricted but only to the extent that the sale and distribution of a device may be restricted under a regulation under section 520(e); and

"(C) shall, where appropriate, require the use and prescribe the form and content of labeling for the proper installation, maintenance, operation, and use of the device.

"(3) A performance standard established under this section may not include any provision not required or authorized by paragraph (2) of this subsection.

"(4) The Secretary shall provide for periodic evaluation of performance standards established under this section to determine if such standards should be changed to reflect new medical, scientific, or other technological data.

"(5) In carrying out his duties under this section, the Secretary shall, to the maximum extent practicable—

"(A) use personnel, facilities, and other technical support available in other Federal agencies,

"(B) consult with other Federal agencies concerned with standard-setting and other nationally or internationally recognized standard-setting entities, and

"(C) invite appropriate participation, through joint or other conferences, workshops, or other means, by informed persons representative of scientific, professional, industry, or consumer organizations who in his judgment can make a significant contribution.

"Initiation of a Proceeding for a Performance Standard

"(b) (1) A proceeding for the development of a performance standard for a device shall be initiated by the Secretary by the publication in the Federal Register of notice of the opportunity to submit to the Secretary a request (within fifteen days of the date of the publication of the notice) for a change in the classification of the device based on new information relevant to its classification.

"(2) If, after publication of a notice pursuant to paragraph (1) the Secretary receives a request for a change in the device's classification, he shall, within sixty days of the publication of such notice and after consultation with the appropriate panel under section 513, by order published in the Federal Register, either deny the request for change in classification or give notice of his intent to initiate such a change under section 513(e).

"Invitation for Standards

"(c) (1) If, after the publication of a notice under subsection (b), no action is required under paragraph (2) of such subsection or the Secretary denies a request to change the classification of the device with respect to which such notice was published, the Secretary shall publish in the Federal Register a notice inviting any person, including any Federal agency, to—

"(A) submit to the Secretary, within sixty days after the date of publication of the notice, an existing standard as a proposed performance standard for such device, or

"(B) offer, within sixty days after the date of publication of the notice, to develop such a proposed standard.

"(2) A notice published pursuant to paragraph (1) for an offer for the development of a proposed performance standard for a device—

"(A) shall specify a period within which the standard is to be developed, which period may be extended by the Secretary for good cause shown; and

"(B) shall include—

"(i) a description or other designation of the device,

"(ii) a statement of the nature of the risk or risks associated with the use of the device and intended to be controlled by a performance standard, "(iii) a summary of the data on which the Secretary has found a need for initiation of the proceeding to develop a performance standard, and

"(iv) identification of any existing performance standard known to the Secretary which may be relevant to the proceeding.

"(3) The Secretary shall by regulation require that an offeror of an offer to develop a proposed performance standard submit to the Secretary such information concerning the offeror as the Secretary determines is relevant with respect to the offeror's qualifications to develop a proposed performance standard for a device, including information respecting the offeror's financial stability, expertise, and experience, and any potential conflicts of interest, including financial interest in the device for which the proposed standard is to be developed, which may be relevant with respect to the offeror's qualifications. Such information submitted by an offeror may not be made public by the Secretary unless required by section 552 of title 5, United States Code.

"(4) If the Secretary determines that a performance standard can be developed by any Federal agency (including an agency within the Department of Health, Education, and Welfare), the Secretary may—

"(A) if such determination is made with respect to an agency within such Department, develop such a standard in lieu of accepting any offer to develop such a standard pursuant to a notice published pursuant to subsection (c), or

"(B) if such determination is made with respect to any other agency, authorize such agency to develop such a standard in lieu of accepting any such offer.

In making such a determination respecting a Federal agency, the Secretary shall take into account the personnel and expertise within such agency. The requirements described in subparagraphs (B) and (C) of subsection (e) (4) shall apply to development of a standard under this paragraph.

"Acceptance of Certain Existing Standards

"(d) (1) If the Secretary—

"(A) determines that a performance standard has been issued or adopted or is being developed by any Federal agency or by any other qualified entity or receives a performance standard submitted pursuant to a notice published pursuant to subsection (c), and

"(B) determines that such performance standard is based upon scientific data and information and has been subjected to scientific consideration,

he may, in lieu of accepting any offer to develop such a standard pursuant to a notice published pursuant to subsection (c), accept such standard as a proposed performance standard for such device or as a basis upon which a proposed performance standard may be developed.

"(2) If a standard is submitted to the Secretary pursuant to a notice published pursuant to subsection (c) and the Secretary does not accept such standard, he shall publish in the Federal Register notice of that fact together with the reasons therefor.

"Acceptance of Offer To Develop Standard

"(e) (1) Except as provided by subsections (c) (4) and (d), the Secretary shall accept one, and may accept more than one, offer to develop a proposed performance standard for a device pursuant to a notice published pursuant to subsection (c) if he determines that (A) the offeror is qualified to develop such a standard and is technically competent to undertake and complete the development of an appropriate performance standard within the period specified in the notice, and (B) the offeror will comply with procedures prescribed by regulations of the Secretary under paragraph (4) of this subsection. In determining the qualifications of an offeror to develop a standard, the Secretary shall take into account the offeror's financial stability, expertise, experience, and any potential conflicts of interest, including financial interest in the device for which such standard is to be developed, which may be relevant with respect to the offeror's qualifications.

"(2) The Secretary shall publish in the Federal Register the name and address of each person whose offer is accepted under paragraph (1) and a summary of the terms of such offer as accepted.

"(3) If such an offer is accepted, the Secretary may, upon application which may be made prior to the acceptance of the offer, agree to contribute to the offeror's cost in developing a proposed standard if the Secretary determines that such contribution is likely to result in a more satisfactory standard than would be developed without such contribution. The Secretary shall by regulation prescribe the items of cost in which he will participate, except that such items may not include the cost of construction (except minor remodeling) or the acquisition of land or buildings. Payments to an offeror under this paragraph may be made without regard to section 3648 of the Revised Statutes (31 U.S.C. 529).

"(4) The Secretary shall prescribe regulations governing the development of proposed standards by persons whose offers are accepted under paragraph (1). Such regulations shall, notwithstanding subsection (b) (A) of section 553 of title 5, United States Code, be promulgated in accordance with the requirements of that section for notice and opportunity for participation and shall—

"(A) require that performance standards proposed for promulgation be supported by such test data or other documents or materials as the Secretary may reasonably require to be obtained;

"(B) require that notice be given to interested persons of the opportunity to participate in the development of such performance standards and require the provision of such opportunity;

"(C) require the maintenance of records to disclose (i) the course of the development of performance standards proposed for promulgation, (ii) the comments and other information submitted by any person in connection with such development, including comments and information with respect to the need for such performance standards, and (iii) such other matters as may be relevant to the evaluation of such performance standards;

"(D) provide that the Secretary and the Comptroller General of the United States, or any of their duly authorized representatives, shall have access for the purpose of audit and examination to any books, documents, papers, and other records, relevant to the expenditure of any funds contributed by the Secretary under paragraph (3); and

"(E) require the submission of such periodic reports as the Secretary may require to disclose the course of the development of performance standards proposed for promulgation.

"(5) If an offer is made pursuant to a notice published pursuant to subsection (c) and the Secretary does not accept such offer, he shall publish in the Federal Register notice of that determination together with the reasons therefor.

"Development of Standard by Secretary After Publication
of Subsection (c) Notice

"(f) If the Secretary has published a notice pursuant to subsection (c) and—

"(1) no person makes an offer or submits a standard pursuant to the notice;

"(2) the Secretary has not accepted an existing performance standard under subsection (d) or accepted an offer to develop a proposed performance standard pursuant to the notice; or

"(3) the Secretary has accepted an offer or offers to develop a proposed performance standard, but determines, thereafter that—

"(A) the offeror under each such offer is unwilling or unable to continue the development of the performance standard which was the subject of the offer or offers, or

"(B) the performance standard which has been developed is not satisfactory, and publishes notice of that determination in the Federal Register together with his reasons therefor;

then the Secretary may proceed to develop a proposed performance standard. The requirements described in subparagraphs (B) and (C) of subsection (e) (4) shall apply to the development of a standard by the Secretary under this subsection.

"Establishment of a Standard

"(g) (1) (A) After publication pursuant to subsection (c) of a notice respecting a performance standard for a device, the Secretary shall either—

"(i) publish, in the Federal Register in a notice of proposed rulemaking, a proposed performance standard for the device (I) developed by an offeror under such notice and accepted by the Secretary, (II) developed under subsection (c) (4), (III) accepted by the Secretary under subsection (d), or (IV) developed by him under subsection (f), or

"(ii) issue a notice in the Federal Register that the proceeding is terminated together with the reasons for such termination.

"(B) If the Secretary issues under subparagraph (A) (ii) a notice of termination of a proceeding to establish a performance standard for a device, he shall (unless such notice is issued because the device is a banned device under section 516) initiate a proceeding under section 513(e) to reclassify the device subject to the proceeding terminated by such notice.

"(2) A notice of proposed rulemaking for the establishment of a performance standard for a device published under paragraph (1) (A) (i) shall set forth proposed findings with respect to the degree of the risk of illness or injury designed to be eliminated or reduced by the proposed standard and the benefit to the public from the device.

"(3) (A) After the expiration of the period for comment on a notice of proposed rulemaking published under paragraph (1) respecting a performance standard and after consideration of such comments and any report from an advisory committee under paragraph (5), the Secretary shall (i) promulgate a regulation establishing a performance standard and publish in the Federal Register findings on the matters referred to in paragraph (2), or (ii) publish a notice terminating the proceeding for the development of the standard together with the reasons for such termination. If a notice of termination is published, the Secretary shall unless such notice is issued because the device is a banned device under section 516 initiate a proceeding under section 513(e) to reclassify the device subject to the proceeding terminated by such notice.

"(B) A regulation establishing a performance standard shall set forth the date or dates upon which the standard shall take effect, but no such regulation may take effect before one year after the date of its publication unless (i) the Secretary determines that an earlier effective date is necessary for the protection of the public health and safety, or (ii) such standard has been established for a device which, effective upon the effective date of the standard, has been reclassified from class III to class II. Such date or dates shall be established so as to minimize, consistent with the public health and safety, economic loss to, and disruption or dislocation of, domestic and international trade.

"(4) (A) The Secretary, upon his own initiative or upon petition of an interested person, may by regulation, promulgated in accordance with the requirements of paragraphs (2) and (3) (B) of this subsection, amend or revoke a performance standard.

"(B) The Secretary may declare a proposed amendment of a performance standard to be effective on and after its publication in the Federal Register and until the effective date of any final action taken on such amendment if he determines, after affording all interested persons an opportunity for an informal hearing, that making it so effective is in the public interest. A proposed amendment of a performance standard made so effective under the preceding sentence may not prohibit, during the period in which it is so effective, the introduction or delivery for introduction into interstate commerce of a device which conforms to such standard without the change or changes provided by such proposed amendment.

"(5) (A) The Secretary—

"(i) may on his own initiative refer a proposed regulation for the establishment, amendment, or revocation of a performance standard, or

"(ii) shall, upon the request of an interested person unless the Secretary finds the request to be without good cause or the request is made after the expiration of the period for submission of comments on such proposed regulation refer such proposed regulation, to an advisory committee of experts, established pursuant to subparagraph (B), for a report and recommendation with respect to any matter involved in the proposed regulation which requires the exercise of scientific judgment. If a proposed regulation is referred under this subparagraph to an advisory committee, the Secretary shall provide the advisory committee with the data and information on which such proposed regulation is based. The advisory committee shall, within sixty days of the referral of a proposed regulation and after independent study of the data and information furnished to it by the Secretary and other data and information before it, submit to the Secretary a report and recommendation respecting such regulation, together with all underlying data and information and a statement of the reasons or basis for the recommendation. A copy of such report and recommendation shall be made public by the Secretary.

"(B) The Secretary shall establish advisory committees (which may not be panels under section 513) to receive referrals under subparagraph (A). The Secretary shall appoint as members of any such advisory committee persons qualified in the subject matter to be referred to the committee and of appropriately diversified professional background, except that the Secretary may not appoint to such a committee any individual who is in the regular full-time employ of the United States and engaged in the administration of this Act. Each such committee shall include as nonvoting members a representative of consumer interests and a representative of interests of the device manufacturing industry. Members of an advisory committee who are not officers or employees of the United States, while attending conferences or meetings of their committee or otherwise serving at the request of the Secretary, shall be entitled to receive compensation at rates to be fixed by the Secretary, which rates may not exceed the daily equivalent of the rate in effect for grade GS-18 of the General Schedule, for each day (including traveltime) they are so engaged; and while so serving away from their homes or regular places of business each member may be allowed travel expenses, including per diem in lieu of subsistence, as authorized by section 5703 of title 5 of the United States Code for persons in the Government service employed intermittently. The Secretary shall designate one of the members of each advisory committee to serve as chairman thereof. The Secretary shall furnish each advisory committee with clerical and other assistance, and shall by regulation prescribe the procedures to be followed by each such committee in acting on referrals made under subparagraph (A).

"PREMARKET APPROVAL
"General Requirement
"Sec. 515. (a) A class III device—
"(1) which is subject to a regulation promulgated under subsection (b); or
"(2) which is a class III device because of section 513(f),
is required to have, unless exempt under section 520(g), an approval under this section of an application for premarket approval.
"Regulation To Require Premarket Approval
"(b) (1) In the case of a class III device which—

"(A) was introduced or delivered for introduction into interstate commerce for commercial distribution on or before the date of enactment of this section; or

"(B) is (i) of a type so introduced or delivered, and (ii) is substantially equivalent to another device within that type,
the Secretary shall by regulation, promulgated in accordance with this subsection, require that such device have an approval under this section of an application for premarket approval.

"(2) (A) A proceeding for the promulgation of a regulation under paragraph (1) respecting a device shall be initiated by the publication in the Federal Register of a notice of proposed rulemaking. Such notice shall contain—

"(i) the proposed regulation;

"(ii) proposed findings with respect to the degree of risk of illness or injury designed to be eliminated or reduced by requiring the device to have an approved application for premarket approval and the benefit to the public from use of the device;

"(iii) opportunity for the submission of comments on the proposed regulation and the proposed findings; and

"(iv) opportunity to request a change in the classification of the device based on new information relevant to the classification of the device.

"(B) If, after publication of a notice under subparagraph (A), the Secretary receives a request for a change in the classification of a device, he shall, after consultation with the appropriate panel under section 513, by order published in the Federal Register either deny the request for change in classification or give notice of his intent to initiate such a change under section 513(e).

"(3) After the expiration of the period for comment on a proposed regulation and proposed findings published under paragraph (2) and after consideration of comments submitted on such proposed regulation and findings, the Secretary shall (A) promulgate such regulation and publish in the Federal Register findings on the matters referred to in paragraph (2) (A) (ii), or (B) publish a notice terminating the proceeding for the promulgation of the regulation together with the reasons for such termination. If a notice of termination is published, the Secretary shall (unless such notice is issued because the device is a banned device under section 516) initiate a proceeding under section 513(e) to reclassify the device subject to the proceeding terminated by such notice.

"(4) The Secretary, upon his own initiative or upon petition of an interested person, may by regulation amend or revoke any regulation promulgated under this subsection. A regulation to amend or revoke a regulation under this subsection shall be promulgated in accordance with the requirements prescribed by this subsection for the promulgation of the regulation to be amended or revoked.

"Application for Premarket Approval

"(c) (1) Any person may file with the Secretary an application for premarket approval for a class III device. Such an application for a device shall contain—

"(A) full reports of all information, published or known to or which should reasonably be known to the applicant, concerning investigations which have been made to show whether or not such device is safe and effective;

"(B) a full statement of the components, ingredients, and properties of the principle or principles of operation, of such device;

"(C) a full description of the methods used in, and the facilities and controls used for, the manufacture, processing, and, when relevant, packing and installation of, such device;

"(D) an identifying reference to any performance standard under section 514 which would be applicable to any aspect of such device if it were a class II device, and either adequate information to show that such aspect of such device fully meets such performance standard or adequate information to justify any deviation from such standard;

"(E) such samples of such device and of components thereof as the Secretary may reasonably require, except that where the submission of such samples is impracticable or unduly burdensome, the requirement of this subparagraph may be met by the submission of complete information concerning the location of one or more such devices readily available for examination and testing;

"(F) specimens of the labeling proposed to be used for such device; and

"(G) such other information relevant to the subject matter of the application as the Secretary, with the concurrence of the appropriate panel under section 513, may require.

"(2) Upon receipt of an application meeting the requirements set forth in paragraph (1), the Secretary shall refer such application to the appropriate panel under section 513 for study and for submission (within such period as he may establish) of a report and recommendation respecting approval of the application, together with all underlying data and the reasons or basis for the recommendation.

"Action on an Application for Premarket Approval

"(d) (1) (A) As promptly as possible, but in no event later than one hundred and eighty days after the receipt of an application under subsection (c) (except as provided in Section 520 (1) (3) (d) (ii) or unless, in accordance with subparagraph (B) (i), an additional period is agreed upon by the Secretary and the applicant), the Secretary, after considering the report and recommendation submitted under paragraph (2) of such subsection, shall—

"(i) issue an order approving the application if he finds that none of the grounds for denying approval specified in paragraph (2) of this subsection applies; or

"(ii) deny approval of the application if he finds (and sets forth the basis for such finding as part of or accompanying such denial) that one or more grounds for denial specified in paragraph (2) of this subsection apply.

"(B) (i) The Secretary may not enter into an agreement to extend the period in which to take action with respect to an application submitted for a device subject to a regulation promulgated under subsection (b) unless he finds that the continued availability of the device is necessary for the public health.

"(ii) An order approving an application for a device may require as a condition to such approval that the sale and distribution of the device be restricted but only to the extent that the sale and distribution of a device may be restricted under a regulation under section 520(e).

"(2) The Secretary shall deny approval of an application for a device if, upon the basis of the information submitted to the Secretary as part of the application and any other information before him with respect to such device, the Secretary finds that—

"(A) there is a lack of a showing of reasonable assurance that such device is safe under the conditions of use prescribed, recommended, or suggested in the proposed labeling thereof;

"(B) there is a lack of a showing of reasonable assurance that the device is effective under the conditions of use prescribed, recommended, or suggested in the proposed labeling thereof;

"(C) the methods used in, and the facilities and controls used for, the manufacture, processing, and packing and installation of such device do not conform to the requirements of section 520(f);

"(D) based on a fair evaluation of all material facts, the proposed labeling is false or misleading in any particular; or

"(E) such device is not shown to conform in all respects to a performance standard in effect under section 514 compliance with which is a condition to approval of the application and there is a lack of adequate information to justify the deviation from such standard.

Any denial of an application shall, insofar as the Secretary determines to be practicable, be accompanied by a statement informing the applicant of the measures required to place such application in approvable form (which measures may include further research by the applicant in accordance with one or more protocols prescribed by the Secretary).

"(3) An applicant whose application has been denied approval may, by petition filed on or before the thirtieth day after the date upon which he receives notice of such denial, obtain review thereof in accordance with either paragraph (1) or (2) of subsection (g), and any interested person may obtain review, in accordance with paragraph (1) or (2) of subsection (g), of an order of the Secretary approving an application.

"Withdrawal of Approval of Application

"(e) (1) The Secretary shall, upon obtaining, where appropriate, advice on scientific matters from a panel or panels under section 513, and after due notice and opportunity for informal hearing to the holder of an approved application for a device, issue an order withdrawing approval of the application if the Secretary finds—

"(A) that such device is unsafe or ineffective under the conditions of use prescribed, recommended, or suggested in the labeling thereof;

"(B) on the basis of new information before him with respect to such device, evaluated together with the evidence available to him when the application was approved, that there is a lack of a showing of reasonable assurance that the device is safe or effective under the conditions of use prescribed, recommended, or suggested in the labeling thereof;

"(C) that the application contained or was accompanied by an untrue statement of a material fact;

"(D) that the applicant (i) has failed to establish a system for maintaining records, or has repeatedly or deliberately failed to maintain records or to make reports, required by an applicable regulation under section 519(a), (ii) has refused to permit access to, or copying or verification of, such records as required by section 704, or (iii) has not complied with the requirements of section 510;

"(E) on the basis of new information before him with respect to such device, evaluated together with the evidence before him when the application was approved, that the methods used in, or the facilities and controls used for, the manufacture, processing, packing, or installation of such device do not conform with the requirements of section 520(f) and were not brought into conformity with such requirements within a reasonable time after receipt of written notice from the Secretary of nonconformity;

"(F) on the basis of new information before him, evaluated together with the evidence before him when the application was approved, that the labeling of such device, based on a fair evaluation of all material facts, is false or misleading in any particular and was not corrected within a reasonable time after receipt of written notice from the Secretary of such fact; or

"(G) on the basis of new information before him, evaluated together with the evidence before him when the application was approved, that such device is not shown to conform in all respects to a performance standard which is in effect under section 514 compliance with which was a condition to approval of the application and that there is a lack of adequate information to justify the deviation from such standard.

"(2) The holder of an application subject to an order issued under paragraph (1) withdrawing approval of the application may, by petition filed on or before the thirtieth day after the date upon which he receives notice of such withdrawal, obtain review thereof in accordance with either paragraph (1) or (2) of subsection (g).

"Product Development Protocol

"(f) (1) In the case of a class III device which is required to have an approval of an application submitted under subsection (c), such device shall be considered as having such an approval if a notice of completion of testing conducted in accordance with a product development protocol approved under paragraph (4) has been declared completed under paragraph (6).

"(2) Any person may submit to the Secretary a proposed product development protocol with respect to a device. Such a protocol shall be accompanied by data supporting it. If, within thirty days of the receipt of such a protocol, the Secretary determines that it appears to be appropriate to apply the requirements of this subsection to the device with respect to which the protocol is submitted, he shall refer the proposed protocol to the appropriate panel under section 513 for its recommendation respecting approval of the protocol.

"(3) A proposed product development protocol for a device may be approved only if—

"(A) the Secretary determines that it is appropriate to apply the requirements of this subsection to the device in lieu of the requirement of approval of an application submitted under subsection (c); and

"(B) the Secretary determines that the proposed protocol provides—

"(i) a description of the device and the changes which may be made in the device,

"(ii) a description of the preclinical trials (if any) of the device and a specification of (I) the results from such trials to be required before the commencement of clinical trials of the device, and (II) any permissible variations in preclinical trials and the results therefrom,

"(iii) a description of the clinical trials (if any) of the device and a specification of (I) the results from such trials to be required before the filing of a notice of completion of the requirements of the protocol, and (II) any permissible variations in such trials and the results therefrom,

"(iv) a description of the methods to be used in, and the facilities and controls to be used for, the manufacture, processing, and, when relevant, packing and installation of the device,

"(v) an identifying reference to any performance standard under section 514 to be applicable to any aspect of such device,

"(vi) if appropriate, specimens of the labeling proposed to be used for such device,

"(vii) such other information relevant to the subject matter of the protocol as the Secretary, with the concurrence of the appropriate panel or panels under section 513, may require, and

"(viii) a requirement for submission of progress reports and, when completed, records of the trials conducted under the protocol which records are adequate to show compliance with the protocol.

"(4) The Secretary shall approve or disapprove a proposed product development protocol submitted under paragraph (2) within one hundred and twenty days of its receipt unless an additional period is agreed upon by the Secretary and the person who submitted the protocol. Approval of a protocol or denial of approval of a protocol is final agency action subject to judicial review under chapter 7 of title 5, United States Code.

"(5) At any time after a product development protocol for a device has been approved pursuant to paragraph (4), the person for whom the protocol was approved may submit a notice of completion—

"(A) stating (i) his determination that the requirements of the protocol have been fulfilled and that, to the best of his knowledge, there is no reason bearing on safety or effectiveness why the notice of completion should not become effective, and (ii) the data and other information upon which such determination was made, and

"(B) setting forth the results of the trials required by the protocol and all the information required by subsection (c) (1).

"(6) (A) The Secretary may, after providing the person who has an approved protocol an opportunity for an informal hearing and at any time prior to receipt of notice of completion of such protocol, issue a final order to revoke such protocol if he finds that—

"(i) such person has failed substantially to comply with the requirements of the protocol,

"(ii) the results of the trials obtained under the protocol differ so substantially from the results required by the protocol that further trials cannot be justified, or

"(iii) the results of the trials conducted under the protocol or available new information do not demonstrate that the device tested under the protocol does not present an unreasonable risk to health and safety.

"(B) After the receipt of a notice of completion of an approved protocol the Secretary shall, within the ninety-day period beginning on the date such notice is received, by order either declare the protocol completed or declare it not completed. An order declaring a protocol not completed may take effect only after the Secretary has provided the person who has the protocol opportunity for an informal hearing on the order. Such an order may be issued only if the Secretary finds—

"(i) such person has failed substantially to comply with the requirements of the protocol,

"(ii) the results of the trials obtained under the protocol differ substantially from the results required by the protocol, or

"(iii) there is a lack of a showing of reasonable assurance of the safety and effectiveness of the device under the conditions of use prescribed, recommended, or suggested in the proposed labeling thereof.

"(C) A final order issued under subparagraph (A) or (B) shall be in writing and shall contain the reasons to support the conclusions thereof.

"(7) At any time after a notice of completion has become effective, the Secretary may issue an order (after due notice and opportunity for an informal hearing to the person for whom the notice is effective) revoking the approval of a device provided by a notice of completion which has become effective as provided in subparagraph (A) if he finds that any of the grounds listed in subparagraphs (A) through (G) of subsection (e) (1) of this section apply. Each reference in such subparagraphs to an application shall be considered for purposes of this paragraph as a reference to a protocol and the notice of completion of such protocol, and each reference to the time when an application was approved shall be considered for purposes of this paragraph as a reference to the time when a notice of completion took effect.

"(8) A person who has an approved protocol subject to an order issued under paragraph (6) (A) revoking such protocol, a person who has an approved protocol with respect to which an order under paragraph (6) (B) was issued declaring that the protocol had not been completed, or a person subject to an order issued under paragraph (7) revoking the approval of a device may, by petition filed on or before the thirtieth day after the date

upon which he receives notice of such order, obtain review thereof in
accordance with either paragraph (1) or (2) of subsection (g).

"Review

"(g) (1) Upon petition for review of—

"(A) an order under subsection (d) approving or denying approval of
an application or an order under subsection (e) withdrawing approval
of an application, or

"(B) an order under subsection (f) (6) (A) revoking an approved
protocol, under subsection (f) (6) (B) declaring that an approved
protocol has not been completed, or under subsection (f) (7) revoking
the approval of a device,

the Secretary shall, unless he finds the petition to be without good cause
or unless a petition for review of such order has been submitted under
paragraph (2), hold a hearing, in accordance with section 554 of title 5 of
the United States Code, on the order. The panel or panels which considered the application, protocol, or device subject to such order shall
designate a member to appear and testify at any such hearing upon request
of the Secretary, the petitioner, or the officer conducting the hearing, but
this requirement does not preclude any other member of the panel or
panels from appearing and testifying at any such hearing. Upon completion of such hearing and after considering the record established in such
hearing, the Secretary shall issue an order either affirming the order
subject to the hearing or reversing such order and, as appropriate, approving or denying approval of the application, reinstating the application's
approval, approving the protocol, or placing in effect a notice of completion.

"(2) (A) Upon petition for review of—

"(i) an order under subsection (d) approving or denying approval
of an application or an order under subsection (e) withdrawing
approval of an application, or

"(ii) an order under subsection (f) (6) (A) revoking an approved
protocol, under subsection (f) (6) (B) declaring that an approved
protocol has not been completed, or under subsection (f) (7) revoking the approval of a device,

the Secretary, unless he is required to provide review of such order under
paragraph (1), shall refer the application or protocol subject to the order
and the basis for the order to an advisory committee of experts established
pursuant to subparagraph (B) for a report and recommendation with
respect to the order. The advisory committee shall, after independent
study of the data and information furnished to it by the Secretary and
other data and information before it, submit to the Secretary a report and
recommendation, together with all underlying data and information and a
statement of the reasons or basis for the recommendation. A copy of such
report shall be promptly supplied by the Secretary to any person who
petitioned for such referral to the advisory committee.

"(B) The Secretary shall establish advisory committees (which may not
be panels under section 513) to receive referrals under subparagraph (A).
The Secretary shall appoint as members of any such advisory committee
persons qualified in the subject matter to be referred to the committee and

of appropriately diversified professional background, except that the Secretary may not appoint to such a committee any individual who is in the regular full-time employ of the United States and engaged in the administration of this Act. Each such committee shall include as nonvoting members a representative of consumer interests and a representative of interests of the device manufacturing industry. Members of an advisory committee (other than officers or employees of the United States), while attending conferences or meetings of their committee or otherwise serving at the request of the Secretary, shall be entitled to receive compensation rates to be fixed by the Secretary, which rates may not exceed the daily equivalent for grade GS-18 of the General Schedule for each day (including traveltime) they are so engaged; and while so serving away from their homes or regular places of business each member may be allowed travel expenses, including per diem in lieu of subsistence, as authorized by section 5703 of title 5 of the United States Code for persons in the Government service employed intermittently. The Secretary shall designate the chairman of an advisory committee from its members. The Secretary shall furnish each advisory committee with clerical and other assistance, and shall by regulation prescribe the procedures to be followed by each such committee in acting on referrals made under subparagraph (A).

"(C) The Secretary shall make public the report and recommendation made by an advisory committee with respect to an application and shall by order, stating the reasons therefor, either affirm the order referred to the advisory committee or reverse such order and, if appropriate, approve or deny approval of the application, reinstate the application's approval, approve the protocol, or place in effect a notice of completion.

"Service of Orders

"(h) Orders of the Secretary under this section shall be served (1) in person by any officer or employee of the department designated by the Secretary, or (2) by mailing the order by registered mail or certified mail addressed to the applicant at his last known address in the records of the Secretary.

"BANNED DEVICES
"General Rule

"Sec. 516. (a) Whenever the Secretary finds, on the basis of all available data and information and after consultation with the appropriate panel or panels under section 513, that—

"(1) a device intended for human use presents substantial deception or an unreasonable and substantial risk of illness or injury; and

"(2) in the case of substantial deception or an unreasonable and substantial risk of illness or injury which the Secretary determines can be corrected or eliminated by labeling or change in labeling, such labeling or change in labeling was not done within a reasonable time after written notice to the manufacturer from the Secretary specifying the deception or risk of illness or injury, the labeling or change in labeling to correct the deception or eliminate or reduce such risk, and the period within which such labeling or change in labeling is to be done;

he may initiate a proceeding to promulgate a regulation to make such device a banned device. The Secretary shall afford all interested persons opportunity for an informal hearing on a regulation proposed under this subsection.

"Special Effective Date

"(b) The Secretary may declare a proposed regulation under subsection (a) to be effective upon its publication in the Federal Register and until the effective date of any final action taken respecting such regulation if (1) he determines, on the basis of all available data and information, that the deception or risk of illness or injury associated with the use of the device which is subject to the regulation presents an unreasonable, direct, and substantial danger to the health of individuals, and (2) before the date of the publication of such regulation, the Secretary notifies the manufacturer of such device that such regulation is to be made so effective. If the Secretary makes a proposed regulation so effective, he shall, as expeditiously as possible, give interested persons prompt notice of his action under this subsection, provide reasonable opportunity for an informal hearing on the proposed regulation, and either affirm, modify, or revoke such proposed regulation.

"JUDICIAL REVIEW
"Application of Section

"Sec. 517. (a) Not later than thirty days after—

"(1) the promulgation of a regulation under section 513 classifying a device in class I or changing the classification of a device to class I or an order under subsection (f) (2) of such section classifying a device or denying a petition for classification of a device,

"(2) the promulgation of a regulation under section 514 establishing, amending, or revoking a performance standard for a device,

"(3) the issuance of an order under section 514 (b) (2) or 515 (b) (2) (B) denying a request for reclassification of a device,

"(4) the promulgation of a regulation under paragraph (3) of section 515 (b) requiring a device to have an approval of a premarket application, a regulation under paragraph (4) of that section amending or revoking a regulation under paragraph (3), or an order pursuant to section 515 (g) (1) or 515 (g) (2) (C),

"(5) the promulgation of a regulation under section 516 (other than a proposed regulation made effective under subsection (b) of such section upon the regulation's publication) making a device a banned device,

"(6) the issuance of an order under section 520 (f) (2), or

"(7) an order under section 520 (g) (4) disapproving an application for an exemption of a device for investigational use or an order under section 520 (g) (5) withdrawing such an exemption for a device,

any person adversely affected by such regulation or order may file a petition with the United States Court of Appeals for the District of Columbia or for the circuit wherein such person resides or has his principal place of business for judicial review of such regulation or order. A copy of the petition shall be transmitted by the clerk of the court to the Secretary or other officer designated by him for that purpose. The Secretary shall

file in the court the record of the proceedings on which the Secretary
based his regulation or order as provided in section 2112 of title 28,'
United States Code. For purposes of this section, the term 'record' means
all notices and other matter published in the Federal Register with respect
to the regulation or order reviewed, all information submitted to the
Secretary with respect to such regulation or order, proceedings of any
panel or advisory committee with respect to such regulation or order, any
hearing held with respect to such regulation or order, and any other
information identified by the Secretary, in the administrative proceeding
held with respect to such regulation or order, as being relevant to such
regulation or order.

"Additional Data, Views, and Arguments

"(b) If the petitioner applies to the court for leave to adduce additional data, views, or arguments respecting the regulation or order being
reviewed and shows to the satisfaction of the court that such additional
data, views, or arguments are material and that there were reasonable
grounds for the petitioner's failure to adduce such data, views, or arguments in the proceedings before the Secretary, the court may order the
Secretary to provide additional opportunity for the oral presentation of
data, views, or arguments and for written submissions. The Secretary may
modify his findings, or make new findings by reason of the additional
data, views, or arguments so taken and shall file with the court such
modified or new findings, and his recommendation, if any, for the modification or setting aside of the regulation or order being reviewed, with the
return of such additional data, views, or arguments.

"Standard for Review

"(c) Upon the filing of the petition under subsection (a) of this section
for judicial review of a regulation or order, the court shall have jurisdiction
to review the regulation or order in accordance with chapter 7 of title 5,
United States Code, and to grant appropriate relief, including interim
relief, as provided in such chapter. A regulation described in paragraph (2)
or (5) of subsection (a) and an order issued after the review provided by
section 515 (g) shall not be affirmed if it is found to be unsupported by
substantial evidence on the record taken as a whole.

"Finality of Judgments

"(d) The judgment of the court affirming or setting aside, in whole or
in part, any regulation or order shall be final, subject to review of the
Supreme Court of the United States upon certiorari or certification, as
provided in section 1254 of title 28 of the United States Code.

"Other Remedies

"(e) The remedies provided for in this section shall be in addition to
and not in lieu of any other remedies provided by law.

"Statement of Reasons

"(f) To facilitate judicial review under this section or under any other
provision of law of a regulation or order issued under section 513, 514,
515, 516, 518, 519, 520, or 521, each such regulation or order shall
contain a statement of the reasons for its issuance and the basis, in the
record of the proceedings held in connection with its issuance, for its
issuance.

"NOTIFICATION AND OTHER REMEDIES
"Notification

"Sec. 518. (a) If the Secretary determines that—

"(1) a device intended for human use which is introduced or delivered for introduction into interstate commerce for commercial distribution presents an unreasonable risk or substantial harm to the public health, and

"(2) notification under this subsection is necessary to eliminate the unreasonable risk of such harm and no more practicable means is available under the provisions of this Act (other than this section) to eliminate such risk,

the Secretary may issue such order as may be necessary to assure that adequate notification is provided in an appropriate form, .by the persons and means best suited under the circumstances involved, to all health professionals who prescribe or use the device and to any other person (including manufacturers, importers, distributors, retailers, and device users) who should properly receive such notification in order to eliminate such risk. An order under this subsection shall require that the individuals exposed to the risk with respect to which the order is to be issued be included in the persons to be notified of the risk unless the Secretary determines that notice to such individuals would present a greater danger to the health of such individuals than no such notification. If the Secretary makes such a determination with respect to such individuals, the order shall require that the health professionals who prescribe or use the device notify the individuals whom the health professionals treated with the device of the risk presented by the device and of any action which may be taken by or on behalf of such individuals to eliminate or reduce such risk. Before issuing an order under this subsection, the Secretary shall consult with the persons who are to give notice under the order.

"Repair, Replacement, or Refund

"(b) (1) (A) If, after affording opportunity for an informal hearing, the Secretary determines that—

"(i) a device intended for human use which is introduced or delivered for introduction into interstate commerce for commercial distribution presents an unreasonable risk of substantial harm to the public health,

"(ii) there are reasonable grounds to believe that the device was not properly designed and manufactured with reference to the state of the art as it existed at the time of its design and manufacture,

"(iii) there are reasonable grounds to believe that the unreasonable risk was not caused by failure of a person other than a manufacturer, importer, distributor, or retailer of the device to exercise due care in the installation, maintenance, repair, or use of the device, and

"(iv) the notification authorized by subsection (a) would not by itself be sufficient to eliminate the unreasonable risk and action described in paragraph (2) of this subsection as necessary to eliminate such risk,

the Secretary may order the manufacturer, importer, or any distributor of such device, or any combination of such persons, to submit to him within a reasonable time a plan for taking one or more of the actions described in paragraph (2). An order issued under the preceding sentence which is directed to more than one person shall specify which person may decide which action shall be taken under such plan and the person specified shall be the person who the Secretary determines bears the principal, ultimate financial responsibility for action taken under the plan unless the Secretary cannot determine who bears such responsibility or the Secretary determines that the protection of the public health requires that such decision be made by a person (including a device user or health professional) other than the person he determines bears such responsibility.

"(B) The Secretary shall approve a plan submitted pursuant to an order issued under subparagraph (A) unless he determines (after affording opportunity for an informal hearing) that the action or actions to be taken under the plan or the manner in which such action or actions are to be taken under the plan will not assure that the unreasonable risk with respect to which such order was issued will be eliminated. If the Secretary disapproves a plan, he shall order a revised plan to be submitted to him within a reasonable time. If the Secretary determines (after affording opportunity for an informal hearing) that the revised plan is unsatisfactory or if no revised plan or no initial plan has been submitted to the Secretary within the prescribed time, the Secretary shall (i) prescribe a plan to be carried out by the person or persons to whom the order issued under subparagraph (A) was directed, or (ii) after affording an opportunity for an informal hearing, by order prescribe a plan to be carried out by a person who is a manufacturer, importer, distributor, or retailer of the device with respect to which the order was issued but to whom the order under subparagraph (A) was not directed.

"(2) The actions which may be taken under a plan submitted under an order issued under paragraph (1) are as follows:

"(A) To repair the device so that it does not present the unreasonable risk of substantial harm with respect to which the order under paragraph (1) was issued.

"(B) To replace the device with a like or equivalent device which is in conformity with all applicable requirements of this Act.

"(C) To refund the purchase price of the device (less a reasonable allowance for use if such device has been in the possession of the device user for one year or more—

"(i) at the time of notification ordered under subsection (a), or

"(ii) at the time the device user receives actual notice of the unreasonable risk with respect to which the order was issued under paragraph (1), whichever first occurs).

"(3) No charge shall be made to any person (other than a manufacturer, importer, distributor, or retailer (who avails himself of any remedy, described in paragraph (2) and provided under an order issued under paragraph (1), and the person subject to the order shall reimburse each person (other than a manufacturer, importer, distributor, or retailer) who is entitled to such a remedy for any reasonable and foreseeable expenses actually incurred by such person in availing himself of such remedy.

"Reimbursement

"(c) An order issued under subsection (b) with respect to a device may require any person who is a manufacturer, importer, distributor, or retailer of the device to reimburse any other person who is a manufacturer, importer, distributor, or retailer of such device for such other person's expenses actually incurred in connection with carrying out the order if the Secretary determines such reimbursement is required for the protection of the public health. Any such requirement shall not affect any rights or obligations under any contract to which the person receiving reimbursement or the person making such reimbursement is a party.

"Effect on Other Liability

"(d) Compliance with an order issued under this section shall not relieve any person from liability under Federal or State law. In awarding damages for economic loss in an action brought for the enforcement of any such liability, the value to the plaintiff in such action of any remedy provided him under such order shall be taken into account.

"RECORDS AND REPORTS ON DEVICES

"General Rule

"Sec. 519. (a) Every person who is a manufacturer, importer, or distributor of a device intended for human use shall establish and maintain such records, make such reports, and provide such information, as the Secretary may by regulation reasonably require to assure that such device is not adulterated or misbranded and to otherwise assure its safety and effectiveness. Regulations prescribed under the preceding sentence—

"(1) shall not impose requirements unduly burdensome to a device manufacturer, importer, or distributor taking into account his cost of complying with such requirements and the need for the protection of the public health and the implementation of this Act;

"(2) which prescribe the procedure for making requests for reports or information shall require that each request made under such regulations for submission of a report or information to the Secretary state the reason or purpose for such request and identify to the fullest extent practicable such report or information;

"(3) which require submission of a report or information to the Secretary shall state the reason or purpose for the submission of such report or information and identify to the fullest extent practicable such report or information;

"(4) may not require that the identity of any patient be disclosed in records, reports, or information required under this subsection unless required for the medical welfare of an individual, to determine the safety or effectiveness of a device, or to verify a record, report, or information submitted under this Act; and

"(5) may not require a manufacturer, importer, or distributor of a class I device to—

"(A) maintain records respecting information not in the possession of the manufacturer, importer, or distributor, or

"(B) to submit to the Secretary any report or information—

"(i) not in the possession of the manufacturer, importer, or distributor, or

"(ii) on a periodic basis,

unless such report or information is necessary to determine if the device should be reclassified or if the device is adulterated or misbranded.

In prescribing such regulations, the Secretary shall have due regard for the professional ethics of the medical profession and the interests of patients. The prohibitions of paragraph (4) of this subsection continue to apply to records, reports, and information concerning any individual who has been a patient, irrespective of whether or when he ceases to be a patient.

"Persons Exempt

"(b) Subsection (a) shall not apply to—

"(1) any practitioner who is licensed by law to prescribe or administer devices intended for use in humans and who manufactures or imports devices solely for use in the course of his professional practice;

"(2) any person who manufactures or imports devices intended for use in humans solely for such person's use in research or teaching and not for sale (including any person who uses a device under an exemption granted under section 520(g)); and

"(3) any other class of persons as the Secretary may by regulation exempt from subsection (a) upon a finding that compliance with the requirements of such subsection by such class with respect to a device is not necessary to (A) assure that a device is not adulterated or misbranded or (B) otherwise to assure its safety, and effectiveness.

"GENERAL PROVISIONS RESPECTING CONTROL OF DEVICES INTENDED FOR HUMAN USE

"General Rule

"Sec. 520. (a) Any requirement authorized by or under section 501, 502, 510, or 519 applicable to a device intended for human use shall apply to such device until the applicability of the requirement to the device has been changed by action taken under section 513, 514, or 515 or under subsection (g) of this section, and any requirement established by or under section 501, 503, 510, or 519 which is inconsistent with a requirement imposed on such device under section 514 or 515 or under subsection (g) of this section shall not apply to such device.

"Custom Devices

"(b) Sections 514 and 515 do not apply to any device which, in order to comply with the order of a physician or dentist (or any other specially qualified person designated under regulations promulgated by the Secretary after an opportunity for an oral hearing) necessarily deviates from an otherwise applicable performance standard or requirement prescribed by or under section 514 or 515 if (1) the device is not generally available in finished form for purchase or for dispensing upon prescription and is not offered through labeling or advertising by the manufacturer, importer, or distributor thereof for commercial distribution, and (2) such device—

"(A) (i) is intended for use by a patient named in such order of such physician or dentist (or other specially qualified person so designated), or

"(ii) is intended solely for use by (I) such physician or dentist (or other specially qualified person so designated) or (II) a person under his professional supervision in the course of the professional practice of such physician or dentist (or other specially qualified person so designated), and

"(B) is not generally available to or generally used by other physicians or dentists (or other specially qualified persons so designated).

"Trade Secrets

"(c) Any information reported to or otherwise obtained by the Secretary or his representative under section 513, 514, 515, 516, 518, 519, or 704 or under subsection (f) or (g) of this section which is exempt from disclosure pursuant to subsection (a) of section 552 of title 5, United States Code, by reason of subsection (b) (4) of such section shall be considered confidential and shall not be disclosed and may not be used by the Secretary as the basis for the reclassification of a device under section 513 from class III to class II or as the basis for the establishment or amendment of a performance standard under section 514 for a device reclassified from class III to class II, except that such information may be disclosed to other officers or employees concerned with carrying out this Act or when relevant in any proceeding under this Act (other than section 513 or 514 thereof).

"Notices and Findings

"(d) Each notice of proposed rulemaking under section 513, 514, 515, 516, 518, or 519, or under this section, any other notice which is published in the Federal Register with respect to any other action taken under any such section and which states the reasons for such action, and each publication of findings required to be made in connection with rulemaking under any such section shall set forth—

"(1) the manner in which interested persons may examine data and other information on which the notice or findings is based, and

"(2) the period within which interested persons may present their comments on the notice or findings (including the need therefor) orally or in writing, which period shall be at least sixty days but may not exceed ninety days unless the time is extended by the Secretary by a notice published in the Federal Register stating good cause therefor.

"Restricted Devices

"(e) (1) The Secretary may by regulation require that a device be restricted to sale or distribution—

"(A) only upon the written or oral authorization of a practitioner licensed by law to administer or use such device, or

"(B) upon such other conditions (other than any condition which would limit the use of a device to a particular category or categories of physicians defined by their training or experience) as the Secretary may prescribe in such regulation,

if, because of its potentiality for harmful effect or the colateral measures necessary to its use, the Secretary determines that there cannot otherwise be reasonable assurance of its safety and effectiveness. A device subject to a regulation under this subsection is a restricted device.

"(2) A restricted device shall be deemed to be misbranded if its label fails to bear such appropriate statements of the restrictions as the Secretary may in such regulation prescribe.

"Good Manufacturing Practice Requirements

"(f) (1) (A) The Secretary may, in accordance with subparagraph (B), prescribe regulations requiring that the methods used in, and the facilities and controls used for, the manufacture, packing, storage, and installation of a device conform to current good manufacturing practice, as prescribed in such regulations, to assure that the device will be safe and effective and otherwise in compliance with this Act.

"(B) Before the Secretary may promulgate any regulation under subparagraph (A) he shall—

"(i) afford the advisory committee established under paragraph (3) an opportunity to submit recommendations to him with respect to the regulation proposed to be promulgated, and

"(ii) afford opportunity for an oral hearing.

The Secretary shall provide the advisory committee a reasonable time to make its recommendation with respect to proposed regulations under subparagraph (A).

"(2) (A) Any person subject to any requirement prescribed by regulations under paragraph (1) may petition the Secretary for an exemption or variance from such requirement. Such a petition shall be submitted to the Secretary in such form and manner as he shall prescribe and shall—

"(i) in the case of a petition for an exemption from a requirement, set forth the basis for the petitioner's determination that compliance with the requirement is not required to assure that the device will be safe and effective and otherwise in compliance with this Act,

"(ii) in the case of a petition for a variance from a requirement, set forth the methods proposed to be used in, and the facilities and controls proposed to be used for, the manufacture, packing, storage, and installation of the device in lieu of the methods, facilities, and controls prescribed by the requirement, and

"(iii) contain such other information as the Secretary shall prescribe.

"(B) The Secretary may refer to the advisory committee established under paragraph (3) any petition submitted under subparagraph (A). The advisory committee shall report its recommendations to the Secretary with respect to a petition referred to it within sixty days of the date of the petition's referral. Within sixty days after—

"(i) the date the petition was submitted to the Secretary under subparagraph (A), or

"(ii) if the petition was referred to an advisory committee, the expiration of the sixty-day period beginning on the date the petition was referred to the advisory committee,

whichever occurs later, the Secretary shall by order either deny the petition or approve it.

"(C) The Secretary may approve—

"(i) a petition for an exemption for a device from a requirement if he determines that compliance with such requirement is not required to assure that the device will be safe and effective and otherwise in compliance with this Act, and

"(ii) a petition for a variance for a device from a requirement if he determines that the methods to be used in, and the facilities and controls to be used for, the manufacture, packing, storage, and installation of the device in lieu of the methods, controls, and facilities prescribed by the requirement are sufficient to assure that the device will be safe and effective and otherwise in compliance with this Act.

An order of the Secretary approving a petition for a variance shall prescribe such conditions respecting the methods used in, and the facilities and controls used for, the manufacture, packing, storing, and installation of the device to be granted the variance under the petition as may be necessary to assure that the device will be safe and effective and otherwise in compliance with this Act.

"(D) After the issuance of an order under subparagraph (B) respecting a petition, the petitioner shall have an opportunity for an informal hearing on such order.

"(3) The Secretary shall establish an advisory committee for the purpose of advising and making recommendations to him with respect to regulations proposed to be promulgated under paragraph (1) (A) and the approval or disapproval of petitions submitted under paragraph (2). The advisory committee shall be composed of 9 members as follows:

"(A) Three of the members shall be appointed from persons who are officers or employees of any State or local government or of the Federal Government.

"(B) Two of the members shall be appointed from persons who are representative of interests of the device manufacturing industry; two of the members shall be appointed from persons who are representative of the interests of physicians and other health professionals; and two of the members shall be representative of the interests of the general public.

Members of the advisory committee who are not officers or employees of the United States, while attending conferences or meetings of the committee or otherwise engaged in its business, shall be entitled to receive compensation at rates to be fixed by the Secretary, which rates may not exceed the daily equivalent of the rate in effect for grade GS-18 of the General Schedule, for each day (including traveltime) they are so engaged; and while so serving away from their homes or regular places of business each member may be allowed travel expenses, including per diem in lieu of subsistence, as authorized by section 5703 of title 5 of the United States Code for persons in the Government service employed intermittently. The Secretary shall designate one of the members of the advisory committee to serve as its chairman. The Secretary shall furnish the advisory committee with clerical and other assistance. Section 14 of the Federal Advisory

Committee Act shall not apply with respect to the duration of the advisory committee established under this paragraph.

"Exemption for Devices for Investigational Use

"(g) (1) It is the purpose of this subsection to encourage, to the extent consistent with the protection of the public health and safety and with ethical standards, the discovery and development of useful devices intended for human use and to that end to maintain optimum freedom for scientific investigators in their pursuit of that purpose.

"(2) (A) The Secretary shall, within the one hundred and twenty-day period beginning on the date of the enactment of this section, by regulation prescribe procedures and conditions under which devices intended for human use may upon application be granted on exemption from the requirements of section 502, 510, 514, 515, 516, 519, or 706 or subsection (e) or (f) of this section or from any combination of such requirements to permit the investigational use of such devices by experts qualified by scientific training and experience to investigate the safety and effectiveness of such devices.

"(B) The conditions prescribed pursuant to subparagraph (A) shall include the following:

"(i) A requirement that an application be submitted to the Secretary before an exemption may be granted and that the application be submitted in such form and manner as the Secretary shall specify.

"(ii) A requirement that the person applying for an exemption for a device assure the establishment and maintenance of such records, and the making of such reports to the Secretary of data obtained as a result of the investigational use of the device during the exemption, as the Secretary determines will enable him to assure compliance with such conditions, review the progress of the investigation, and evaluate the safety and effectiveness of the device.

"(iii) Such other requirements as the Secretary may determine to be necessary for the protection of the public health and safety.

"(C) Procedures and conditions prescribed pursuant to subparagraph (A) for an exemption may appropriately vary depending on (i) the scope and duration of clinical testing to be conducted under such exemption, (ii) the number of human subjects that are to be involved in such testing, (iii) the need to permit changes to be made in the device subject to the exemption during testing conducted in accordance with a clinical testing plan required under paragraph (3) (A), and (iv) whether the clinical testing of such device is for the purpose of developing data to obtain approval for the commercial distribution of such device.

"(3) Procedures and conditions prescribed pursuant to paragraph (2) (A) shall require, as a condition to the exemption of any device to be the subject of testing involving human subjects, that the person applying for the exemption—

"(A) submit a plan for any proposed clinical testing of the device and a report of prior investigations of the device (including, where appropriate, tests on animals) adequate to justify the proposed clinical testing—

"(i) to the local institutional review committee which has been established in accordance with regulations of the Secretary to supervise clinical testing of devices in the facilities where the proposed clinical testing is to be conducted, or

"(ii) to the Secretary, if—

"(I) no such committee exists, or

"(II) the Secretary finds that the process of review by such committee is inadequate (whether or not the plan for such testing has been approved by such committee),

for review for adequacy to justify the commencement of such testing; and, unless the plan and report are submitted to the Secretary, submit to the Secretary a summary of the plan and a report of prior investigations of the device (including, where appropriate, tests on animals);

"(B) promptly notify the Secretary (under such circumstances and in such manner as the Secretary prescribes) of approval by a local institutional review committee of any clinical testing plan submitted to it in accordance with subparagraph (A);

"(C) in the case of a device to be distributed to investigators for testing, obtain signed agreements from each of such investigators that any testing of the device involving human subjects will be under such investigator's supervision and in accordance with subparagraph (D) and submit such agreements to the Secretary; and

"(D) assure that informed consent will be obtained from each human subject (or his representative) of proposed clinical testing involving such device, except where, subject to such conditions as the Secretary may prescribe, the investigator conducting or supervising the proposed clinical testing of the device determines in writing that there exists a life threatening situation involving the human subject of such testing which necessitates the use of such device and it is not feasible to obtain informed consent from the subject and there is not sufficient time to obtain such consent from his representative.

The determination required by subparagraph (D) shall be concurred in by a licensed physician who is not involved in the testing of the human subject with respect to which such determination is made unless immediate use of the device is required to save the life of the human subject of such testing and there is not sufficient time to obtain such concurrence.

"(4) (A) An application, submitted in accordance with the procedures prescribed by regulations under paragraph (2), for an exemption for a device (other than an exemption from section 516) shall be deemed approved on the thirtieth day after the submission of the application to the Secretary unless on or before such day the Secretary by order disapproves the application and notifies the applicant of the disapproval of the application.

"(B) The Secretary may disapprove an application only if he finds that the investigation with respect to which the application is submitted does not conform to procedures and conditions prescribed under regulations under paragraph (2). Such a notification shall contain the order of disapproval and a complete statement of the reasons for the Secretary's disapproval of the application and afford the applicant opportunity for an informal hearing on the disapproval order.

"(5) The Secretary may by order withdraw an exemption granted under this subsection for a device if the Secretary determines that the conditions applicable to the device under this subsection for such exemption are not met. Such an order may be issued only after opportunity for an informal hearing, except that such an order may be issued before the provision of an opportunity for an informal hearing if the Secretary determines that the continuation of testing under the exemption with respect to which the order is to be issued will result in an unreasonable risk to the public health.

"Release of Safety and Effectiveness Information

"(h) (1) The Secretary shall promulgate regulations under which a detailed summary of information respecting the safety and effectiveness of a device which information was submitted to the Secretary and which was the basis for—

"(A) an order under section 515 (d) (1) (A) approving an application for premarket approval for the device or denying approval of such an application or an order under section 515(e) withdrawing approval of such an application for the device,

"(B) an order under section 515 (f) (6) (A) revoking an approved protocol for the device, an order under section 515 (f) (6) (B) declaring a protocol for the device completed or not completed, or an order under section 515 (f) (7) revoking the approval of the device, or

"(C) an order approving an application under subsection (g) for an exemption for the device from section 516 or an order disapproving, or withdrawing approval of, an application for an exemption under such subsection for the device,

shall be made available to the public upon issuance of the order. Summaries of information made available pursuant to this paragraph respecting a device shall include a summary of any information respecting adverse effects on health of the device.

"(2) The Secretary shall promulgate regulations under which each advisory committee established under section 515 (g) (2) (B) shall make available to the public a detailed summary of information respecting the safety and effectiveness of a device which information was submitted to the advisory committee and which was the basis for its recommendation to the Secretary made pursuant to section 515 (g) (2) (A). A summary of information upon which such a recommendation is based shall be made available pursuant to this paragraph only after the issuance of the order with respect to which the recommendation was made and each such summary shall include a summary of any information respecting the adverse effects on health of the device subject to such order.

"(3) Any information respecting a device which is made available pursuant to paragraph (1) or (2) of this subsection may not be used to establish the safety or effectiveness of another device for purposes of this Act by any person other than the person who submitted the information so made available.

"Proceedings of Advisory Panels and Committees
"(i) Each advisory panel under section 513 and each advisory committee established under section 514(g) (5) (B) or section 515(g) shall made and maintain a transcript of any proceeding of the panel or committee. Each such panel and committee shall delete from any transcript made pursuant to this subsection information which under subsection (c) of this section is to be considered confidential.

"Traceability Requirements
"(j) No regulation under this Act may impose on a type or class of device requirements for the traceability of such type or class of device unless such requirements are necessary to assure the protection of the public health.

"Research and Development
"(k) The Secretary may enter into contracts for research, testing, and demonstrations respecting devices and may obtain devices for research, testing, and demonstration purposes without regard to sections 3648 and 3709 of the Revised Statutes (31 U.S.C. 529, 41 U.S.C. 5).

"Transitional Provisions for Devices Considered as New
Drugs or Antibiotic Drugs
"(l) (1) Any device intended for human use—
"(A) for which on the date of enactment of the Medical Device Amendments of 1975 (hereinafter in this subsection referred to as the 'enactment date') an approval of an application submitted under section 505(b) was in effect;
"(B) for which such an application was filed on or before the enactment date and with respect to which application no order of approval or refusing to approve had been issued on such date under subsection (c) or (d) of such section;
"(C) for which on the enactment date an exemption under subsection (i) of such section was in effect;
"(D) which is within a type of device described in subparagraph (A), (B), or (C) and is substantially equivalent to another device within that type;
"(E) which the Secretary in a notice published in the Federal Register before the enactment date has declared to be a new drug subject to section 505; or
"(F) with respect to which on the enactment date an action is pending in a United States court under section 302, 303, or 304 for an alleged violation of a provision of section 301 which enforces a requirement of section 505 or for an alleged violation of section 505(a),
is classified in class III unless the Secretary in response to a petition submitted under paragraph (2) has classified such device in class I or II.
"(2) The manufacturer or importer of a device classified under paragraph (1) may petition the Secretary (in such form and manner as he shall prescribe) for the issuance of an order classifying the device in class I or class II. Within thirty days of the filing of such a petition, the Secretary shall notify the petitioner of any deficiencies in the petition which prevent the Secretary from making a decision on the petition. Except as provided

in paragraph (3) (D) (ii), within one hundred and eighty days after the filing of a petition under this paragraph and after affording the petitioner an opportunity for an informal hearing, the Secretary shall, after consultation with the appropriate panel under section 513, by order either deny the petition or order the classification, in accordance with the criteria prescribed by section 513 (a) (1) (A) or 513 (a) (1) (B), of the device in class I or class II.

"(3) (A) In the case of a device which is described in paragraph (1) (A) and which is in class III—

"(i) such device shall on the enactment date be considered a device with an approved application under section 515, and

"(ii) the requirements applicable to such device before the enactment date under section 505 shall continue to apply to such device until changed by the Secretary as authorized by this Act.

"(B) In the case of a device which is described in paragraph (1) (B) and which is in class III, an application for such device shall be considered as having been filed under section 515 on the enactment date. The period in which the Secretary shall act on such application in accordance with section 515 (d) (1) shall be one hundred and eighty days (or such greater period as the Secretary and the applicant may agree upon after the Secretary has made the finding required by section 515 (d) (1) (B) (i)) less the number of days in the period beginning on the date an application for such device was filed under section 505 and ending on the enactment date. After the expiration of such period such device is required, unless exempt under subsection (g), to have in effect an approved application under section 515.

"(C) A device which is described in paragraph (1) (C) and which is in class III shall be considered a new drug until the expiration of the ninety-day period beginning on the date of the promulgation of regulations under subsection (g) of this section. After the expiration of such period such device is required, unless exempt under subsection (g), to have in effect an approved application under section 515.

"(D) (i) Except as provided in clause (ii), a device which is described in subparagraph (D), (E), or (F) of paragraph (1) and which is in class III is required to have on and after the enactment date in effect an approved application under section 515.

"(ii) If—

"(I) a petition is filed under paragraph (2) for a device described in subparagraph (D), (E), or (F) of paragraph (1), or

"(II) an application for premarket approval is filed under section 515 for such a device,

within the sixty-day period beginning on the enactment date (or within such greater period as the Secretary, after making the finding required under section 515 (d) (1) (B), and the petitioner or applicant may agree upon), the Secretary shall act on such petition or application in accordance with paragraph (2) or section 515 except that the period within which the Secretary must act on the petition or application shall be within the one hundred and twenty-day period beginning on the date the petition or application is filed. If such a petition or application is filed within such sixty-day (or greater) period, clause (i) of this subparagraph shall not apply to such device before the expiration of such one hundred and twenty-day period, or if such petition is denied or such application is denied approval, before the date of such denial, whichever occurs first.

"(4) Any device intended for human use which on the enactment date was subject to the requirements of section 507 shall be subject to such requirements as follows:

"(A) In the case of such a device which is classified into class I, such requirements shall apply to such device until the effective date of the regulation classifying the device into such class.

"(B) In the case of such a device which is classified into class II, such requirements shall apply to such device until the effective date of a performance standard applicable to the device under section 514.

"(C) In the case of such a device which is classified into class III, such requirements shall apply to such device until the date on which the device is required to have in effect an approved application under section 515.

"STATE AND LOCAL REQUIREMENTS RESPECTING DEVICES
"General Rule

"Sec. 521. (a) Except as provided in subsection (b), no State or political subdivision of a State may establish or continue in effect with respect to a device intended for human use any requirement—

"(1) which is different from, or in addition to, any requirement applicable under this Act to the device, and

"(2) which relates to the safety or effectiveness of the device or to any other matter included in a requirement applicable to the device under this Act.

"Exempt Requirements

"(b) Upon application of a State or a political subdivision thereof, the Secretary may, by regulation promulgated after notice and opportunity for an oral hearing, exempt from subsection (a), under such conditions as may be prescribed in such regulation, a requirement of such State or political subdivision applicable to a device intended for human use if—

"(1) the requirement is more stringent than a requirement under this Act which would be applicable to the device if an exemption were not in effect under this subsection; or

"(2) the requirement—

"(A) is required by compelling local conditions, and

"(B) compliance with the requirement would not cause the device to be in violation of any applicable requirement under this Act."

CONFORMING AMENDMENTS
Amendments to Section 201

Sec. 3. (a) (1) (A) Paragraph (h) of section 201 is amended to read as follows:

"(h) (1) The term 'device' (except when used in paragraph (n) of this section and in sections 301(i), 403(f), 502(c), and 602(c)) means an instrument, apparatus, implement, machine, contrivance, implant, in vitro reagent, or other similar or related article, including any component, part, or accessory, which is—

"(1) recognized in the official National Formulary, or the United States Pharmacopeia, or any supplement to them,

"(2) intended for use in the diagnosis of disease or other conditions, or in the cure, mitigation, treatment, or prevention of disease, in man or other animals, or

"(3) intended to affect the structure or any function of the body of man or other animals, and

which does not achieve any of its principal intended purposes through chemical action within or on the body of man or other animals and which is not dependent upon being metabolized for the achievement of any of its principal intended purposes."

(B) Section 15(d) of the Federal Trade Commission Act is amended to read as follows:

"(d) The Term 'device' (except when used in subsection (a) of this section) means an instrument, apparatus, implement, machine, contrivance, implant, in vitro reagent, or other similar or related article, including any component, part, or accessory, which is—

"(1) recognized in the official National Formulary, or the United States Pharmacopeia, or any supplement to them,

"(2) intended for use in the diagnosis of disease or other conditions, or in the cure, mitigation, treatment, or prevention of disease, in man or other animals, or

"(3) intended to affect the structure or any function of the body of man or other animals, and

which does not achieve any of its principal intended purposes through chemical action within or on the body of man or other animals and which is not dependent upon being metabolized for the achievement of any of its principal intended purposes.".

(2) Section 201 is amended by adding at the end the following:

"(y) The term 'informal hearing' means a hearing which is not subject to section 554, 556, or 557 of title 5 of the United States Code and which provides for the following:

"(1) The presiding officer in the hearing shall be designated by the Secretary from officers and employees of the Department of Health, Education, and Welfare who have not participated in any action of the Secretary which is the subject of the hearing and who are not directly responsible to an officer or employee of the Department who has participated in any such action.

"(2) Each party to the hearing shall have the right at all times to be advised and accompanied by an attorney.

"(3) Before the hearing, each party to the hearing shall be given reasonable notice of the matters to be considered at the hearing, including a comprehensive statement of the basis for the action taken or proposed by the Secretary which is the subject of the hearing and a general summary of the information which will be presented by the Secretary at the hearing in support of such action.

"(4) At the hearing the parties to the hearing shall have the right to hear a full and complete statement of the action of the Secretary which is the subject of the hearing together with the information and reasons supporting such action, to conduct reasonable questioning, and to present any oral or written information relevant to such action.

"(5) The presiding officer in such hearing shall prepare a written report of the hearing to which shall be attached all written material presented at the hearing. The participants in the hearing shall be given the opportunity to review and correct or supplement the presiding officer's report of the hearing.

"(6) The Secretary may require the hearing to be transcribed. A party to the hearing shall have the right to have the hearing transcribed at his expense. Any transcription of a hearing shall be included in the presiding officer's report of the hearing.".

Amendments to Section 301

(b) (1) Section 301 is amended by adding at the end the following new paragraphs:

"(q) (1) The failure or refusal to (A) comply with any requirement prescribed under section 518 or 520(g), or (B) furnish any notification or other material or information required by or under section 519 or 520(g).

"(2) With respect to any device, the submission of any report that is required by or under this Act that is false or misleading in any material respect.

"(r) The introduction or delivery for introduction into interstate commerce for export of a device or drug in violation of an order issued under section 801(d) (7).".

(2) Section 301(e) is amended by striking out "or" before "512" and by inserting after "(m)" a comma and the following: "515(f), or 519".

(3) Section 301(j) is amended by inserting "510," before "512", by inserting "513, 515, 514, 516, 518, 519, 520(g)," before "704," and by striking out "or 706" and inserting in lieu thereof "706, or 707".

(4) Section 301(1) is amended (A) by inserting "or device" after "drug" each time it occurs, and (B) by striking out "505" and inserting in lieu thereof "505, 515, or 520(g), as the case may be".

Amendments to Section 304

(c) Section 304(a) is amended (1) by striking out "device," in paragraph (1), and (2) by striking out "and" before "(C)" in paragraph (2), and (3) by striking out the period at the end of that paragraph and inserting in lieu thereof a comma and the following: "and (D) any adulterated or misbranded device.".

Amendments to Section 501

(d) Section 501 is amended by adding at the end the following new paragraphs:

"(e) If it is, or purports to be or is represented as, a device which is subject to a performance standard established under section 514, unless such device is in all respects in conformity with such standard.

"(f) (1) If it is a class III device—

"(A) (i) which is required by a regulation promulgated under subsection (b) of section 515 to have an approval under such section of an application for premarket approval and which is not exempt from section 515 under section 520(g), and

"(ii) (I) for which an application for premarket approval or a notice of completion of a product development protocol was not filed with the Secretary within the ninety-day period beginning on the date of the promulgation of such regulation, or

"(II) for which such an application was filed and approval of the application has been denied or withdrawn, or such a notice was filed and has been declared not completed or the approval of the device under the protocol has been withdrawn;

"(B) (i) which was initially classified under section 513(f) into class III, which under section 515(a) is required to have an approval of an application for premarket approval, and which is not exempt from section 515 under section 520(g), and

"(ii) which does not have an approval under section 515 of an application for premarket approval; or

"(C) which was initially classified under section 520(l) into class III, which under such section is required to have in effect an approved application under section 515, and which does not have such an application in effect.

"(2) (A) In the case of a device initially classified under section 513(f) into class III and intended solely for investigational use, paragraph (1) (B) shall not apply with respect to such device during the period ending on the ninetieth day after the date of the promulgation of the regulations prescribing the procedures and conditions required by section 520 (g) (2).

"(B) In the case of a device subject to a regulation promulgated under subsection (b) of section 515, paragraph (1) shall not apply with respect to such device during the period ending—

"(i) on the last day of the thirtieth calendar month beginning after the month in which the classification of the device in class III became effective under section 513, or

"(ii) on the ninetieth day after the date of the promulgation of such regulation,

whichever occurs later.

"(g) If it is a banned device.

"(h) If it is a device and the methods used in, or the facilities or controls used for, its manufacture, packing, storage, or installation are not in conformity with applicable requirements under section 520 (f) (1) or an applicable condition prescribed by an order under section 520 (f) (2).

"(i) If it is a device for which an exemption has been granted under section 520(g) for investigational use and the person who was granted such exemption or any investigator who uses such device under such exemption fails to comply with a requirement prescribed by or under such section.".

Amendments to Section 502

(e) (1) Section 502 is amended by adding at the end the following new paragraphs:

"(q) In the case of any restricted device distributed or offered for sale in any State, if (1) its advertising is false or misleading in any particular, or

(2) it is sold or otherwise distributed in violation of regulations prescribed under section 520(e).

"(r) In the case of any restricted device distributed or offered for sale in any State, unless the manufacturer, packer, or distributor thereof includes in all advertisements and other descriptive printed matter issued or caused to be issued by the manufacturer, packer, or distributor with respect to that device (1) a true statement of the device's established name as defined in section 502(e), printed prominently and in type at least half as large as that used for any trade or brand name thereof, and (2) a brief statement of the intended uses of the device and relevant warnings, precautions, side effects, and contraindications and, in the case of specific devices made subject to a finding by the Secretary after notice and opportunity for comment that such action is necessary to protect the public health, a full description of the components of such device or the formula showing quantitatively each ingredient of such device to the extent required in regulations which shall be issued by the Secretary after an opportunity for a hearing. Except in extraordinary circumstances, no regulation issued under this paragraph shall require prior approval by the Secretary of the content of any advertisement and no advertisement of a restricted device, published after the effective date of this paragraph shall, with respect to the matters specified in this paragraph or covered by regulations issued hereunder, be subject to the provisions of section 12 through 15 of the Federal Trade Commission Act (15 U.S.C. 52-55). This paragraph shall not be applicable to any printed matter which the Secretary determines to be labeling as defined in section 201(m).

"(s) If it is a device subject to a performance standard established under section 514, unless it bears such labeling as may be prescribed in such performance standard.

"(t) If it is a device and there was a failure or refusal (1) to comply with any requirement prescribed under section 518 respecting the device, or (2) to furnish any notification or other material or information required by or under section 519 respecting the device.".

(2) Section 502(j) is amended by inserting "or manner" after "dosage".

Amendments to Section 801

(f) (1) Section 801(d) is amended to read as follows:

"(d) (1) A food, drug, device, or cosmetic intended for export shall not be deemed to be adulterated or misbranded under this Act if it—

"(A) accords to the specifications of the foreign purchaser,

"(B) is not in conflict with the laws of the country to which it is intended for export,

"(C) is labeled on the outside of the shipping package that it is intended for export, and

"(D) is not sold or offered for sale in domestic commerce.

"(2) Paragraph (1) does not apply to any device which does not comply with an applicable requirement of section 514 or 515 or which is a banned device under section 516 unless, in addition to the requirements of paragraph (1), the device meets the following requirements:

"(A) If the device is intended for export to a country which has an appropriate health agency to review the device and authorize or approve it as safe for its intended use (including investigational use) within such country, such device may be exported to such country only if—

"(i) the device is so reviewed and authorized or approved by such agency, and

"(ii) notification with respect to the export of the device has been provided the Secretary in accordance with paragraph (6).

"(B) If the device is intended for export to a country which does not have an agency described in subparagraph (A), such device may be exported to such country only if the Secretary determines, upon application and after provision to the applicant of opportunity for an informal hearing on the application, that the exportation of the device to such country is not contrary to public health and safety.

"(3) Paragraph (1) does not apply to an antibiotic drug for which a regulation or release is not in effect pursuant to section 507 unless in addition to the requirements of paragraph (1), the drug meets the following requirements:

"(A) If the drug is intended for export to a country which has an appropriate health agency to review the drug and authorize or approve it as safe for its intended use (including investigational use) within such country, such drug may be exported to such country only if—

"(i) the drug is so reviewed and authorized or approved by such agency, and

"(ii) notification with respect to the export of the drug has been provided the Secretary in accordance with paragraph (6).

"(B) If the drug is intended for export to a country which does not have an agency described in subparagraph (A), such drug may be exported to such country only if the Secretary determines, upon application and after provision to the applicant of opportunity for an informal hearing on the application, that the exportation of the drug to such country is not contrary to public health and safety.

"(4) Paragraph (1) does not apply to a new animal drug, or an animal feed bearing or containing a new animal drug, which is unsafe within the meaning of section 512 unless, upon application to make that paragraph apply to such a drug or feed, the Secretary determines, after providing notice and opportunity for an informal hearing on the application, that—

"(A) the drug or feed meets the requirements of paragraph (1),

"(B) its exportation is not contrary to public health and safety of persons within the United States, and

"(C) (i) the appropriate health agency of the country to which the drug or feed is to be exported has reviewed it and authorized or approved it as safe for its intended use (including investigational use) in such country, or

"(ii) if there is no such agency, its exportation to such country is not contrary to public health and safety.

"(5) Notwithstanding section 301(d), a new drug for which an application is not in effect pursuant to section 505 may be introduced or delivered for introduction into interstate commerce for export if the new drug meets the following requirements:

"(A) The drug meets the requirements of paragraph (1).

"(B) If the drug is intended for export to a country which has an appropriate health agency to review the drug and authorize or approve it as safe for its intended use (including investigational use) within such country, such drug may be exported to such country only if—

"(i) the drug is so reviewed and authorized or approved by such agency, and

"(ii) notification with respect to the export of the drug has been provided the Secretary in accordance with paragraph (6).

"(C) If the drug is intended for export to a country which does not have an agency described in subparagraph (A), such drug may be exported to such country only if the Secretary determines, upon application and after provision to the applicant of opportunity for an informal hearing on the application, that the exportation of the drug to such country is not contrary to public health and safety.

"(6) (A) Each person who is required to register under section 510 and who proposes to introduce or deliver for introduction into interstate commerce for export—

"(i) any device which does not comply with an applicable requirement of section 514 or 515 or which is a banned device under section 516,

"(ii) any antibiotic drug for which a regulation or release is not in effect pursuant to section 507, or

"(iii) any new drug for which an application is not in effect pursuant to section 505,

shall, on an annual basis and in accordance with regulations prescribed by the Secretary submit to the Secretary the notice prescribed by subparagraph (B) if the country to which such device or drug is intended for export has an appropriate health agency to review the drug or device and to authorize or approve it as safe for its intended use (including investigational use) in such country. A notice pursuant to this subparagraph may be amended in accordance with regulations of the Secretary.

"(B) The notice required by subparagraph (A) shall—

"(i) identify each drug and device described in subparagraph (A) which is to be introduced or delivered for introduction into interstate commerce for export during the twelve-month period beginning thirty days after the date the notice is submitted,

"(ii) identify the countries to which each such drug and device will be exported, and

"(iii) demonstrate to the satisfaction of the Secretary that each such device and drug complies with the requirements of subparagraph (1) and has been reviewed by the appropriate health agency of the country to which it is being exported and such agency has authorized or approved it as safe for its intended use (including investigational use) in such country.

"(7) The Secretary may, after providing notice and opportunity for informal hearing, issue an order prohibiting the introduction or delivery for introduction in interstate commerce for export of any—

"(A) device which does not comply with an applicable requirement of section 514 or 515 or which is a banned device under section 516,

"(B) antibiotic drug for which a regulation or release is not in effect pursuant to section 507, or

"(C) new drug for which an application is not in effect pursuant to section 505,

if the country to which the device or drug is intended for export has an appropriate health agency to review the device or drug and authorize or approve it as safe for its intended use (including investigational use) within such country and if the Secretary determines that the export of such device or drug is inconsistent with the health and safety of persons within the United States.".

(2) Section 801 (a) (1) is amended by inserting after "conditions" the following: "or, in the case of a device, the methods used in, and the facilities and controls used for, the manufacture, processing, and packing and installation of the device do not conform to the requirements of section 520(f)".

REGISTRATION OF DEVICE MANUFACTURERS

Sec. 4. (a) Section 510 is amended as follows:

(1) The section heading is amended by inserting "AND DEVICES" after "DRUGS".

(2) Subsection (a) (1) is amended by inserting "or device package" after "drug package"; by inserting "or device" after "the drug"; and by inserting "or user" after "consumer".

(3) Subsections (b), (c), and (d) are amended by inserting "or a device or devices" after "drugs" each time it occurs.

(4) Subsection (e) is amended by adding at the end the following: "The Secretary may by regulation prescribe a uniform system for the identification of devices intended for human use and may require that persons who are required to list such devices pursuant to subsection (j) shall list such devices in accordance with such system.".

(5) Subsection (g) is amended by inserting "or devices" after "drugs" each time such term occurs in paragraphs (1), (2), and (3) of such subsection.

(6) Subsection (h) is amended by inserting after "704 and" the following: "every such establishment engaged in the manufacture, propagation, compounding, or processing of a drug or drugs or of a device or devices classified in class II or III".

(7) The first sentence of subsection (i) is amended by inserting ", or a device or devices," after "drug or drugs"; and the second sentence of such subsection is amended by inserting "shall require such establishment to provide the information required by subsection (j) in the case of a device

or devices and" immediately before "shall include" and by inserting "or devices" after "drugs."

(8) Subsection (j) is amended—

(A) in the matter preceding subparagraph (A) of paragraph (1), by striking out "a list of all drugs (by established name" and inserting in lieu thereof "a list of all drugs and a list of all devices and a brief statement of the basis for believing that each device included in the list is a device rather than a drug (with each drug and device in each list listed by its established name", and by striking out "drugs filed" and inserting in lieu thereof "drugs or devices filed";

(B) in paragraph (1) (A), by striking out "such list" and inserting in lieu thereof "the applicable list"; by inserting "or a device intended for human use contained in the applicable list with respect to which a performance standard has been established under section 514 or which is subject to section 515," after "512,"; and by inserting "or device" after "such drug" each time it appears;

(C) in paragraph (1) (B), by striking out "drug contained in such list" before clause (i) and inserting in lieu thereof "drug or device contained in a applicable list";

(D) by amending clause (i) of paragraph (1) (B) to read as follows—

"(i) which drug is subject to section 503(b) (1), or which device is a restricted device, a copy of all labeling for such drug or device, a representative sampling of advertisements for such drug or device, and, upon request made by the Secretary for good cause, a copy of all advertisements for a particular drug product or device, or";

(E) by amending clause (ii) of paragraph (1) (B) to read as follows:

"(ii) which drug is not subject to section 503 (b) (1) or which device is not a restricted device, the label and package insert for such drug or device and a representative sampling of any other labeling for such drug or device;";

(F) in paragraph (1) (C), by striking out "such list" and inserting "an applicable list" in lieu thereof;

(G) in paragraph (1) (D), by striking out "the list" and inserting in lieu thereof "a list"; by inserting "or the particular device contained in such list is not subject to a performance standard established under section 514 or to section 515 or is not a restricted device" after "512,"; and by inserting "or device" after "particular drug product"; and

(H) in paragraph (2), by inserting "or device" after "drug" each time it appears and, in paragraph (2) (C), by inserting "each" before "by established name".

(9) Such section is amended by adding after subsection (j) the following new subsection:

"(k) Each person who is required to register under this section and who proposes to begin the introduction or delivery for introduction into interstate commerce for commercial distribution of a device intended for human use shall, at least ninety days before making such introduction or delivery, report to the Secretary (in such form and manner as the Secretary shall by regulation prescribe)—

"(1) the class in which the device is classified under section 513 or if such person determines that the device is not classified under such section, a statement of that determination and the basis for such person's determination that the device is or is not so classified, and

"(2) action taken by such person to comply with requirements under section 514 or 515 which are applicable to the device.".

(b) (1) Section 301(p) is amended by striking out "510(j)," and inserting in lieu thereof "510(j) or 510(k),".

(2) Section 502(o) is amended (A) by striking out "is a drug and" and (B) by inserting before the period a comma and the following: "if it was not included in a list required by section 510(j), if a notice or other information respecting it was not provided as required by such section or section 510(k), or if it does not bear such symbols from the uniform system for identification of devices prescribed under section 510(e) as the Secretary by regulation requires".

(3) The second sentence of section 801(a) is amended by inserting "or devices" after "drugs" each time it occurs.

DEVICE ESTABLISHED AND OFFICIAL NAMES

Sec. 5. (a) (1) Subparagraph (1) of section 502(e) is amended by striking out "subparagraph (2)" and inserting in lieu thereof "subparagraph (3)".

(2) Subparagraph (2) of such section is redesignated as subparagraph (3) and is amended by striking out "this paragraph (e)" and inserting in lieu thereof "subparagraph (1)".

(3) Such section is amended by adding after subparagraph (1) the following new subparagraph:

"(2) If it is a device and it has an established name, unless its label bears, to the exclusion of any other nonproprietary name, its established name (as defined in paragraph (4)) prominently printed in type at least half as large as that used thereon for any proprietary name or designation for such device, except that to the extent compliance with the requirements of this subparagraph is impracticable, exemptions shall be established by regulations promulgated by the Secretary.".

(4) Such section is amended by adding after subparagraph (3) (as so redesignated) the following:

"(4) As used in subparagraph (2), the term 'established name' with respect to a device means (A) the applicable official name of the device designated pursuant to section 508, (B) if there is no such name and such device is an article recognized in an official compendium, then the official title thereof in such compendium, or (C) if neither clause (A) nor clause (B) of this subparagraph applies, then any common or usual name of such device.".

"(b) Section 508 is amended (1) in subsections (a) and (e) by adding "or device" after "drug" each time it appears; (2) in subsection (b) by adding after "all supplements thereto," the following: "and at such times as he may deem necessary shall cause a review to be made of the official names by which devices are identified in any official compendium (and all supplements thereto)"; (3) in subsection (c) (2) by adding "or device" after "single drug", and by adding "or to two or more devices which are substantially equivalent in design and purpose" after "purity,"; (4) in subsection (c) (3) by adding "or device" after "useful drug", and after "drug or drugs" each time it appears; and (5) in subsection (d) by adding "or devices" after "drugs".

INSPECTIONS RELATING TO DEVICES

Sec. 6. (a) The second sentence of subsection (a) of section 704 (21 U.S.C. 374) is amended by inserting "or restricted devices" after "prescription drugs" both times it appears.

(b) The third sentence of such subsection is amended to read as follows: "No inspection authorized by the preceding sentence shall extend to financial data, sales data other than shipment data, pricing data, personnel data (other than data as to qualifications of technical and professional personnel performing functions subject to this Act, and research data (other than data relating to new drugs, antibiotic drugs, and devices and subject to reporting and inspection under regulations lawfully issued pursuant to section 505(i) or (j), section 507(d) or (g), section 519, or 520(g), and data relating to other drugs or devices which in the case of a new drug would be subject to reporting or inspection under lawful regulations issued pursuant to section 505(j))."

(c) (1) Paragraph (1) of the sixth sentence of such subsection is amended by inserting "or devices" after "drugs" each time it occurs.

(2) Paragraph (2) of that sentence is amended by inserting ",or prescribe or use devices, as the case may be," after "administer drugs"; and by inserting "or, manufacture or process devices," after "process drugs".

(3) Paragraph (3) of that sentence is amended by inserting ", or manufacture or process devices," after "process drugs".

(d) Section 704 is amended by adding at the end the following new subsection:

"(e) Every person required under section 519 or 520(g) to maintain records and every person who is in charge or custody of such records shall, upon request of an officer or employee designated by the Secretary, permit such officer or employee at all reasonable times to have access to, and to copy and verify, such records."

ADMINISTRATIVE RESTRAINT

Sec. 7. (a) Section 304 is amended by adding at the end the following new subsection:

"(g) (1) If during an inspection conducted under section 704 of a facility or a vehicle, a device which the officer or employee making the inspection has reason to believe is adulterated or misbranded is found in such facility or vehicle, such officer or employee may order the device detained (in accordance with regulations prescribed by the Secretary) for a reasonable period which may not exceed twenty days unless the Secretary determines that a period of detention greater than twenty days is required to institute an action under subsection (a) or section 302, in which case he may authorize a detention period of not to exceed thirty days. Regulations of the Secretary prescribed under this paragraph shall require that before a device may be ordered detained under this paragraph the Secretary or an officer or employee designated by the Secretary approve such order. A detention order under this paragraph may require the labeling or marking of a device during the period of its detention for the purpose of identifying the device as detained. Any person who would be entitled to claim a device if it were seized under subsection (a) may appeal to the Secretary a detention of such device under this paragraph. Within five days of the date an appeal of a detention is filed with the Secretary, the Secretary shall after affording opportunity for an informal hearing by order confirm the detention or revoke it.

"(2) (A) Except as authorized by subparagraph (B), a device subject to a detention order issued under paragraph (1) shall not be moved by any person from the place at which it is ordered detained until—

"(i) released by the Secretary, or

"(ii) the expiration of the detention period applicable to such order, whichever occurs first.

"(B) A device subject to a detention order under paragraph (1) may be moved—

"(i) in accordance with regulations prescribed by the Secretary, and

"(ii) if not in final form for shipment, at the discretion of the manufacturer of the device for the purpose of completing the work required to put it in such form."

(b) Section 301 is amended by adding after the paragraph added by section 3 (b) (1) the following new paragraph:

"(s) The movement of a device in violation of an order under section 304(g) or the removal or alteration of any mark or label required by the order to identify the device as detained."

CONFIDENTIAL INFORMATION; PRESUMPTION

Sec. 8. Chapter 7 is amended by adding at the end the following new sections:

"CONFIDENTIAL INFORMATION

"Sec. 707. The Secretary may provide any information which is exempt from disclosure pursuant to subsection (a) of section 552 of title 5, United States Code, by reason of subsection (b) (4) of such section to a person other than an officer or employee of the Department if the Secretary determines such other person requires the information in connection with an activity which is undertaken under contract with the Secretary, which relates to the administration of this Act, and with respect to which the Secretary (or an officer or employee of the Department) is not prohibited from using such information. The Secretary shall require as a condition to the provision of information under this section that the person receiving it take such security precautions respecting the information as the Secretary may by regulation prescribe.

"PRESUMPTION

"Sec. 708. In any action to enforce the requirements of this Act respecting a device the connection with interstate commerce required for jurisdiction in such action shall be presumed to exist.".

COLOR ADDITIVES

Sec. 9. (a) Section 706 is amended (1) by inserting "or device" after "drug" each time it occurs, (2) by inserting "or devices" after "drugs" each time it occurs, and (3) by adding at the end of subsection (a) the following new sentences: "A color additive for use in or on a device shall be subject to this section only if the color additive comes in direct contact with the body of man or other animals for a significant period of time. The Secretary may by regulation designate the uses of color additives in or on devices which are subject to this section.".

(b) (1) Section 501(a) is amended (A) by inserting "(3) if its" in lieu of "(3) if it is a drug and its"; (2) by inserting "(4) if (A) it bears or contains" in lieu of "(4) if (A) it is a drug which bears or contains"; and (3) by inserting "or devices" after "drugs" in subclause (B) of clause (4).

(2) Section 502(m) is amended by striking out "in or on drugs".

ASSISTANCE FOR SMALL MANUFACTURERS OF DEVICES

Sec. 10. The Secretary of Health, Education, and Welfare shall establish within the Department of Health, Education, and Welfare an identifiable office to provide technical and other nonfinancial assistance to small manufacturers of medical devices to assist them in complying with the requirements of the Food, Drug, and Cosmetic Act, as amended by this Act.

APPENDIX B

SUMMARY OF PROPOSED ANSI STANDARDS

John C. Sinclair

This summary is a condensation of the proposed American National Standard for Specification of Hearing Aid characteristics, using as much as possible the language of the proposal. This standard represents the combined work of a highly qualified group of individuals under the most capable leadership and guidance of Samuel F. Lybarger. The membership of ANSI Working Group S3-48 is:

Richard Brander
Mahlon D. Burkhard
Edwin D. Burnett
G. Donald Causey, Ph.D.
William G. Ely
Michael S. Gluck
W. F. S. Hopmeier
James F. Jerger, Ph.D.
Roger N. Kasten, Ph.D.
Hugh S. Knowles
Samuel F. Lybarger
Arthur F. Niemoeller, Ph.D.
James A. Nunley
Wayne O. Olsen, Ph.D.
David A. Preves
John C. Sinclair, Ph.D.
Gerald A. Studebaker, Ph.D.
Harry Teder

The procedures of this standard differ from existing standards in the establishment of a reference test gain-control position to which the hearing aid is adjusted for certain measurements, such as frequency response, harmonic distortion and equivalent input noise level. The reference test gain-control position considers that the gain-control setting for certain tests should be related to the saturation output capability of the hearing aid.

A somewhat different reference test gain-control setting method was originated by the National Bureau of Standards for the Veterans Administration. A random noise signal with a long time average spectrum distribution resembling speech is used to produce a 60 dB sound pressure level in the free field where the hearing aid is placed. The hearing aid gain control is set to produce an output 12 dB below saturation sound pressure level with this signal. Because of the difficulties that have been found in accurately reproducing the specified random noise spectrum in a variety of hearing aid testing systems, including "sound boxes," a pure tone averaging method that is capable of providing accurate measurements and reproducibility in existing measurement systems has been substituted for the random noise method. It has been found to give results very close to those obtained with an accurately shaped random noise signal.

This standard is limited to the specification of electroacoustical characteristics. It is felt that further study is required before standard test procedures relating to mechanical and environmental performance can be established.

DEFINITIONS OF SOME TERMS

Saturation sound pressure level for 90 dB input sound pressure level. The sound pressure level developed in a 2-cm^3 earphone coupler when the input sound pressure level at the microphone sound entrace on the hearing aid is 90 dB SPL with the gain control of the hearing aid full-on. The abbreviation for this term is SSPL90. *Note:* It is recognized that the true saturation level may occur with more, or less, input sound pressure level than 90 dB. However, the differences are usually small over the frequency range of interest and the single input sound pressure level of 90 dB makes automatic recording of the SSPL90 curve very simple.

High-frequency-average saturation sound pressure level. The average of the 1,000, 1,600 and 2,500 Hz values of SSPL90. The abbreviation for the term is HF-average SSPL90. *Note:* The prefix "HF" is used to differentiate this quantity from the "output" as defined in S3.8-1967 (R-1971), which uses 500, 1,000, and 2,000 Hz for averaging.

High-frequency-average full-on gain. The average of the 1,000, 1,600 and 2,500 Hz values of full-on gain. The abbreviation for the term is HF-average full-on gain.

Reference test gain control position. The setting of the hearing aid gain control so that the average of the earphone coupler sound pressure levels at 1,000, 1,600 and 2,500 Hz, with a pure-tone input sound pressure level of 60 dB is 17 dB less than the HF-average SSPL90, or, if the gain available will not permit this, the full-on gain-control position of the hearing aid.

TEST EQUIPMENT

General

The test equipment described in this section conforms in many respects to the requirements for measurements described in American National Standard S3.3-1960 (R-1971). Details are added where necessary for the additional tests or test conditions required in this standard. In particular, the standard considers the input sound pressure level as that at the microphone opening of the hearing aid instead of that in free field as in S3.3-1960 (R-1971).

Recommended Measurements, Specifications, and Tolerances

The results obtained by the methods specified below express the performance under the conditions of the test, but will not generally agree with the performance of the hearing aid under actual conditions of use. The difference between actual and test conditions must be borne in mind in interpreting the test results. In the area of gain, particularly, the use of higher frequencies for averaging will usually give a higher number than the S3.8-1967 (R-1971) or HAIC gain.

Curves

It is recommended that all published curves of gain, response or output versus frequency be plotted on a grid having a linear decibel ordinate scale and a logarithmic frequency abcissa scale with the length of one decade on the abcissa equal to the length of 50 ± 3 decibels on the ordinate.

SSPL90 curve

With the gain control full-on and with basic settings of controls, record or otherwise develop a curve of coupler sound pressure level versus frequency over the range 200–5,000 Hz, using a constant input sound pressure level of 90 dB.

From the above curve, determine the maximum sound pressure level. The maximum sound pressure level as determined shall not exceed that specified by the manufacturer.

HF-average SSPL90

Average the 1,000, 1,600, and 2,500 Hz SSPL90 values.

Tolerance

The HF-average SSPL90 shall be within ± 4 dB of the manufacturer's specified value for the model.

Full-on Gain

Full-on gain shall be measured with the gain control of the hearing aid set to its full-on position and with a sinusoidal input sound pressure level of 60 dB, or, if necessary to maintain linear input-output conditions, with an input sound pressure level of 50 dB. For AGC aids, the input sound pressure level shall be 50 dB. The input sound pressure level shall be stated. The full-on gain is the difference between the coupler sound pressure level and the input sound pressure level.

HF-average Full-on Gain

Average the 1,000, 1,600 and 2,500 Hz full-on gain values.

Tolerance   The HF-average full-on gain shall be within ± 5 dB of the manufacturer's specified value for the model.

Adjustment of the gain control to the reference test position: with an input sound pressure level of 60 dB, adjust the gain control so that the average of the 1,000, 1,600, and 2,500 Hz values of the coupler sound pressure level equals the HF-average SSPL90 minus 17 dB, within ± 1 dB.

If the aid does not have enough gain to permit this adjustment, set the gain control full-on. For AGC aids, set the gain control full-on. *Note:* The long term average sound pressure level for speech at one meter approximates 65 dB. Speech peaks are usually 12 dB above the average level. By adjusting the gain control to give a coupler sound pressure level 12 dB below the saturation level for a 65 dB input sound pressure level, a very rough estimate can be made that speech peaks should not exceed the saturation sound pressure level available in an aid. The use of 60 dB input sound pressure level and a 17 dB gain control setback from the SSPL90 value gives essentially the identical setting, but simplifies measurement with generally used test equipment.

Frequency Response Curve

With the gain control in the reference test position, and with an input sound pressure level of 60 dB, record or otherwise develop the frequency response curve over the range 200–5,000 Hz or a lesser range determined by limits 20 dB below the average of the 1,000, 1,600, and 2,500 Hz response levels. For AGC aids and input sound pressure level of 50 dB is to be employed.

Tolerance Method for Frequency Response Curve

Tolerance range   The following procedure shall be used:
a) From the manufacturer's specified frequency response curve determine the average of the 1,000, 1,600 and 2,500 Hz response levels.
b) Subtract 20 dB.
c) Draw a line parallel to the abcissa at the reduced level.
d) Note the lowest frequency, f_1, at which the response curve intersects the straight line.
e) Note the highest frequency, f_2, at which the response curve intersects the straight line, if this is less than 5,000 Hz.

Frequency range   For information purposes, but not for tolerance purposes, the frequency range of the hearing aid shall be considered as being between f_1 and f_2 (even if f_2 exceeds 5,000 Hz).

Tolerance   The tolerances in two bands shall be as follows:

	Frequency limits	Tolerance
Low band . . .	1.25 f_1 to 2,000 Hz	± 4 dB
High band . . .	2,000 to 4,000 Hz or 0.8f_2, whichever is lower	± 6 dB

Compliance with the tolerances may be determined using a suitable template with upper and lower limits that are derived from the manufacturer's specified response curve for the model. Vertical adjustment of the template on the response curve of the measured hearing aid is permitted. Horizontal adjustment up to 10% in frequency is permitted. Following these adjustments, the entire portion of the curve between 1.25 f_1 and 4,000 Hz or 0.8 f_2, if lower than 4,000 Hz, must lie between the upper and lower limit curves.

Harmonic Distortion

With the gain control in the reference test position and with an input sound pressure level of 70 dB, measure and record the total harmonic distortion in the coupler output for input frequencies of 500, 800 and 1,600 Hz. In the event the response curve rises 12 dB or more between any distortion test frequency and its second harmonic, distortion tests at that test frequency may be omitted.

Equivalent Input Noise Level (L_n)

With the gain control in the test reference position, determine the average of the coupler sound pressure levels at 1,000, 1,600 and 2,500 Hz for an input sound pressure level of 60 dB (L_{ave}). Remove the acoustic signal and record the sound pressure level in the coupler caused by inherent noise (L_2). Then $L_n = L_2 - (L_{ave} - 60)$ dB.

Battery Current

With the gain control in the reference test position, measure the battery current with a pure-tone 1,000 Hz input signal at a sound pressure level of 65 dB.

Coupler Sound Pressure Level with Induction Coil

With the gain control full-on and the hearing aid set to the "T" (telephone input) mode, the hearing aid is placed in an alternating magnetic field having a frequency of 1,000 Hz and a magnetic field strength of 10mA/m and oriented to produce the greatest coupler sound pressure level. This sound pressure level is recorded.

Tolerance   The measured value of the coupler sound pressure level shall be within ± 6 dB of the manufacturer's specified value for test conditions.

AUTOMATIC GAIN CONTROL HEARING AIDS

The following tests apply to AGC aids.

Input-Output Characteristics

Using a pure tone test frequency of 2,000 Hz, measure the coupler sound pressure level for input sound pressure levels from 50 to 90 dB, in 10 dB steps. Plot the coupler sound pressure level along the ordinate against the corresponding input sound pressure level along the abcissa on a grid having linear decibel scales with equal-sized divisions for both ordinate and abcissa. With the measured and specified curves matched at the point corresponding to 70 dB input sound pressure level, the measured curve at 50 dB and 90 dB input sound pressure levels shall not differ in output sound pressure level from the specified curve by more than ± 4 dB.

Dynamic AGC Characteristics

With the gain control full-on and using a square wave modulated pure tone input signal of 2,000 Hz, which alternates abruptly between sound pressure levels of 55 and 80 dB, determine the attack and release times from an oscilloscope pattern. The attack time is defined as the time between the abrupt increase from 55 to 80 dB and the point where the level has stabilized to within 2 dB of the steady state value for the 80 dB input sound pressure level. The release time is defined as the interval between the abrupt drop from 80 to 55 dB and the point where the signal has stabilized to within 2 dB of the steady state value for the 55 dB input sound pressure level.

Tolerance

The attack time and the release time shall each be within ± 5 ms or ± 50%, whichever is larger, of the values specified by the manufacturer for the model.

Interpretation of tolerances The tolerances apply to the performance of the hearing aid as determined with perfectly accurate measurement equipment. To ensure that performance is within a specified tolerance when using imperfect measurement equipment, the tolerance on the measured value must be less than the specified tolerance by the maximum error of measurement. To be sure that performance is outside of the specified tolerance when using imperfect measurement equipment, the tolerance on the measured value must be greater than the specified tolerance by the maximum error of measurement.

INDEX